Atlas of Skin Cancers

Ali Hendi · Juan-Carlos Martinez

Atlas of Skin Cancers

Practical Guide to Diagnosis and Treatment

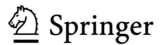

Authors
Ali Hendi, MD
Consultant, Department of Dermatology
Mayo Clinic, Jacksonville, FL
USA
Assistant Professor of Dermatology
College of Medicine
Mayo Clinic, Rochester, MN
USA

Present address:
Private Practice
Chevy Chase, MD
USA
mohsmd@yahoo.com

Juan-Carlos Martinez, MD
Senior Associate Consultant,
Department of Dermatology
Mayo Clinic, Jacksonville, FL
USA
Assistant Professor of Dermatology
College of Medicine
Mayo Clinic, Rochester, MN
USA
martinez.juancarlos@mayo.edu

ISBN 978-3-642-13398-5   e-ISBN 978-3-642-13399-2
DOI 10.1007/978-3-642-13399-2
Springer Heidelberg Dordrecht London New York

Library of Congress Control Number: 2010937910

Cover design: eStudioCalamar, Figueres/Berlin

Printed on acid-free paper

Springer is part of Springer Science+Business Media (www.springer.com)

To my wife Azadeh for her relentless encouragement and faith in me, my parents, Ahmad and Afsar, for their continual support, and Drs. John Zitelli and David Brodland, for their mentorship.

Ali Hendi

To my wife Mary Ellen for her constant love and support, and our beautiful children Carolina and Lucca who have enriched my life in a way I could never have imagined.
To my parents Carlos and Maria Carolina for instilling in me the desire to achieve.
To my mentors Clark Otley, and Jonathan L Cook, for directing my ambitions toward the fascinating world of Mohs surgery and cutaneous oncology.

Juan-Carlos Martinez

Preface

The incidence of skin cancer has risen drastically in recent years. This increase, combined with relatively limited access to specialists in dermatology, leads to many of these patients presenting to their primary care providers with suspicious skin lesions. Even with formal training in dermatology, distinguishing one scaly bump from another with certainty can be quite difficult. This atlas is intended for those providers who wish to sharpen their clinical acumen.

Our aim is to help the reader realize that each entity can have a variety of clinical presentations and should be distinguished, if possible, from a number of mimickers. To that end, we have organized the atlas into separate chapters dedicated to the most common cutaneous malignancies. We provide several examples of each entity and various images of common mimickers. For each entity, we discuss treatment options and provide high-quality clinical images detailing these treatments in a step-by-step fashion.

We must alert the reader that while we wish to provide a visual foundation for many providers, this atlas should not serve as a diagnostic tool; a biopsy is always indicated if the practitioner has any doubt as to the clinical diagnosis. Cutaneous malignancies can be very destructive and, in some cases, fatal if not managed properly. Diagnosis and proper treatment is paramount.

We hope that the readers of this atlas will come away from it better able to serve the needs of their patients.

Chevy Chase, MD, USA   Ali Hendi
Jacksonville, FL, USA   Juan-Carlos Martinez

Acknowledgments

The authors would like to acknowledge the efforts of the following in preparing this atlas:

- Department of Dermatology, Mayo Clinic, Jacksonville, Florida, for providing academic support
- The Section of Medical Photography staff for their expertise
- Donald P. Lookingbill, MD, former Chairman, Department of Dermatology at Mayo Clinic, Jacksonville, Florida, for reviewing the initial outline of the atlas and providing thoughtful feedback
- Ms. M. Alice McKinney for the medical illustrations

Contents

Introduction

1

The skin is the largest organ of the body. A basic understanding of the anatomy of the skin is needed for the proper diagnosis and management of skin cancers. The basic subunits of the skin include the epidermis, dermis, and subcutis (Fig. 1.1). The epidermis is the outermost layer of the skin. The innermost layer of the epidermis is the basal layer. The basal layer cells multiply to form the squamous layer of the epidermis. The outer layer of epidermis is the stratum corneum, which is composed of keratin. Melanocytes (pigment-producing cells) lie within the basal layer of the epidermis. The dermis incorporates the adnexal structures (hair follicles, sebaceous glands, and sweat glands) and is made up of collagen, elastic tissue, and reticular fibers. The subcutis is made up of adipose tissue.

There are terms used in describing skin lesions that are unique to dermatology. This terminology is helpful in documenting lesions and in communicating with colleagues. The basic terminology and associated illustrations are explained in Figs. 1.2–1.7.

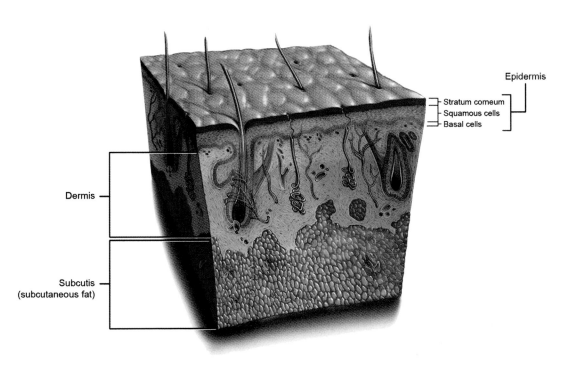

Fig. 1.1
Schematic detailing the multiple layers of the skin

A. Hendi and J.C. Martinez, *Atlas of Skin Cancers*,
DOI: 10.1007/978-3-642-13399-2_1, © Mayo Foundation for Medical Education and Research 2011

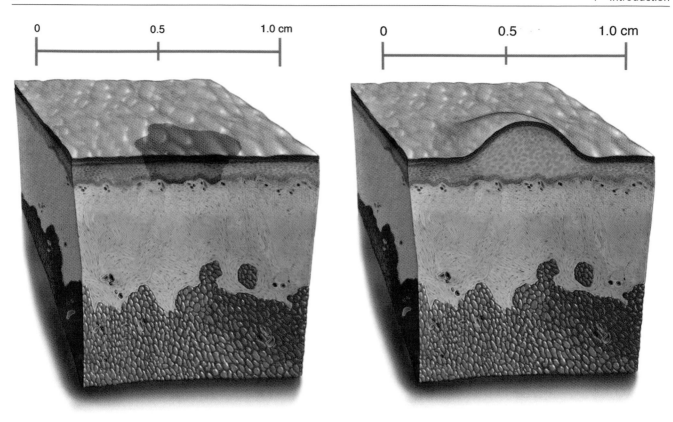

Fig. 1.2
Macule-Flat, <5 mm, circumscribed skin discoloration that lacks surface elevation or depression

Fig. 1.4
Papule-Elevated, solid lesion, <0.5 cm in diameter

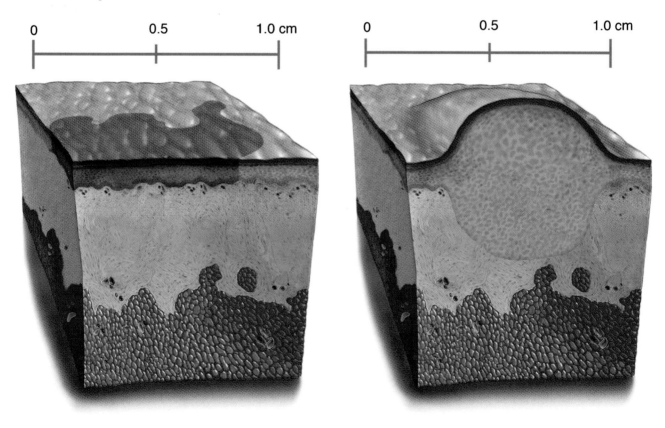

Fig. 1.3
Patch-Flat, >5 mm, circumscribed skin discoloration; a large macule

Fig. 1.5
Plaque-Elevated, flat-topped, solid lesion, >0.5 cm in diameter

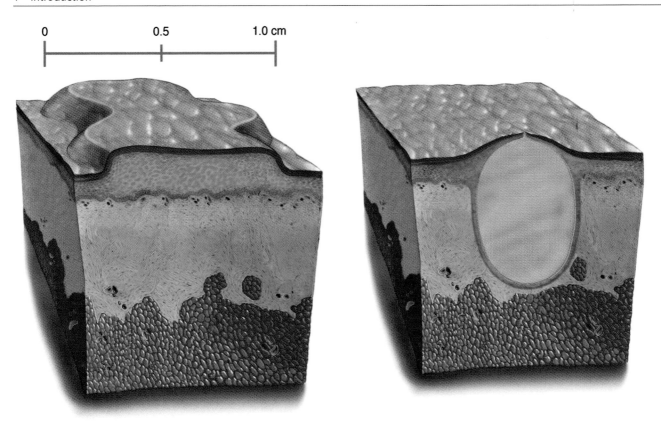

Fig. 1.6
Nodule-Elevated, circular or domed, solid lesion; >0.5 cm in diameter; a large papule

Fig. 1.7
Cyst, a well-circumscribed nodule that has an epithelial lining; generally has a punctum or connection to the surface

Actinic Keratosis

2

2.1 Introduction

While actinic keratoses (AKs) are commonly considered to represent a "premalignant" condition, some authors have asserted that these, in fact, represent the earliest stage of squamous cell carcinoma (SCC) (Ackerman and Mones 2006). Nevertheless, the majority of clinicians do not treat these as malignancies but as precursor lesions with malignant potential. Very common in older, photodamaged patients, they appear as gritty, scaly, pink plaques that are often easier to feel than see. For this reason, palpation of the skin is important in their detection.

Actinic keratoses that become persistent or hypertrophic may evolve into squamous cell carcinoma, and, therefore, they are usually treated. Diagnosis is most commonly made based on clinical appearance. Questionable lesions, or those that fail to respond to initial treatments, should be biopsied to rule out squamous cell carcinoma.

2.2 Treatment of Actinic Keratoses

There are a number of methods available to satisfactorily treat actinic keratoses. Many actinic keratoses will spontaneously clear, and it is not unreasonable to manage conservatively with observation. This modality is best suited for reliable patients that are seen on a routine basis. As the progression of AK to SCC tends to occur rather slowly, observation may be well suited for patients with a decreased life expectancy. While the focus of this atlas is on skin cancer, for the sake of completeness, some of the most commonly used treatment methods for actinic keratoses are covered below.

A. Hendi and J.C. Martinez, *Atlas of Skin Cancers*,
DOI: 10.1007/978-3-642-13399-2_2, © Mayo Foundation for Medical Education and Research 2011

2.2.1 Cryotherapy

Cryotherapy is most commonly used for the treatment of actinic keratoses. This technique usually involves the use of a specialized device that can very precisely control the flow of liquid nitrogen. It is important to recognize that while this technique can be very effective in the destruction of epidermal lesions, it is commonly accompanied by blistering, erosion, and can frequently result in a hypopigmented or depressed scar. Therefore, great care must be taken in limiting the amount of damage to the surrounding tissue, especially in more cosmetically sensitive areas such as the face.

It is critical to realize that studies detailing the use of cryosurgery for the treatment of skin cancers are describing a different technique than that mentioned above. Cryosurgery for skin cancer is a carefully controlled technique whereby thermal sensors are placed in the skin allow for precisely controlled temperatures at specific depths within the tissue. This technique is not commonly employed and should not be confused with the more straightforward spraying of actinic keratoses with liquid nitrogen (Figs. 2.1–2.6).

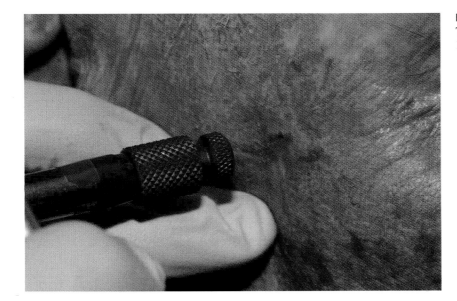

Fig. 2.1
The cryotherapy device is held approximately 1–2 cm from lesion to be treated

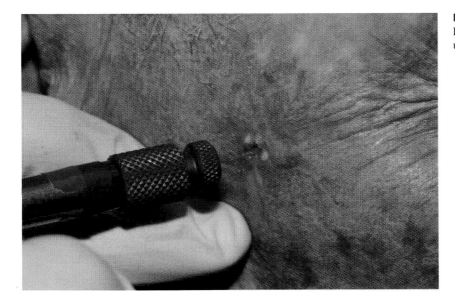

Fig. 2.2
Frost can be noted on skin surface immediately upon commencement of treatment

Fig. 2.3
The frozen area can be seen to expand while spraying continues

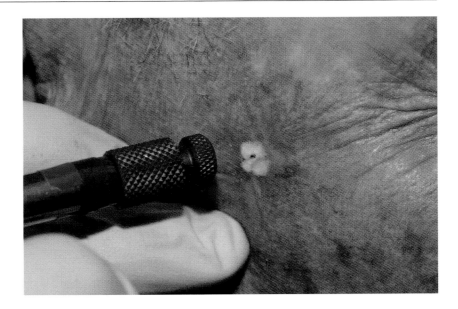

Fig. 2.4
Once the entire area is noted be completely frosted, spraying is discontinued

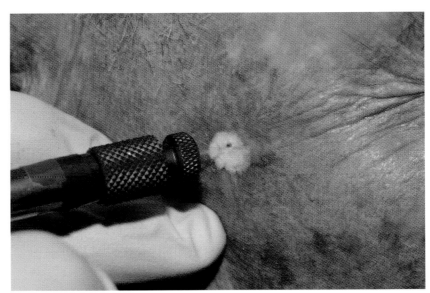

Fig. 2.5
The lesion is noted to thaw slowly after spraying is discontinued

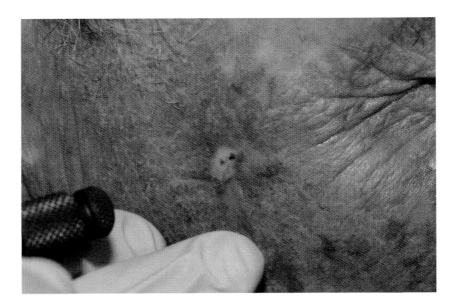

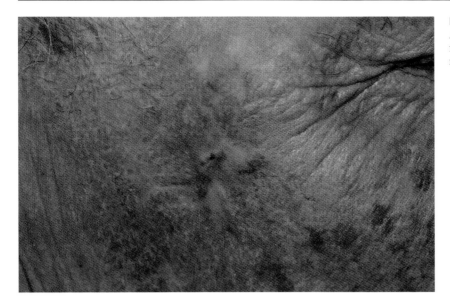

Fig. 2.6
After the frosted area has thawed completely, the freeze–thaw cycle is repeated one to two times more for complete treatment

2.2.2 Topical Treatments

Recent pharmacologic advances have been made for the advent of topical, less invasive treatments for actinic keratoses. These include photodynamic therapy (PDT) and topical creams, such as 5-fluorouracil and imiquimod.

Creams such as imiquimod and 5-fluorouracil (5-FU) have enjoyed great popularity in the treatment of actinic keratoses. These are more commonly employed in the so-called "field treatment" of large areas of sun-damaged skin with numerous AKs. Cure rates for AKs vary depending on the strength of 5-FU used, as well as the duration of the treatment course, but a recent meta-analysis of the effectiveness of 5-FU in the treatment of actinic keratoses suggested that patients can expect an 80–90% reduction in lesions and half of patients can expect complete clearance of all their AKs (Askew et al. 2009).

PDT incorporates the application of a photosensitizing agent followed by irradiation with laser or filtered light. The photosensitizer is applied topically to a selected "field," for example, the forehead and temples, and is preferentially taken up into precancerous or cancerous cells. The area is then treated with light that is absorbed by the photosensitizing molecule, leading to selective destruction of the targeted cells. A variety of photosensitizing agents and light sources has been studied and reviewed, showing modest results in the treatment of actinic keratoses (Tierney et al. 2009). Due to the recent development and continued evolution of PDT, much of the data represent initial clearance rates for particular studies, and excitement should be tempered until long-term cure rates are available and verified.

2.3 Clinical Images of Actinic Keratoses

Fig. 2.7
Diagnosis: Actinic Keratoses-Diffuse
Clinical Description: Diffuse, pink, scaly papules coalescing into
larger plaques on the face

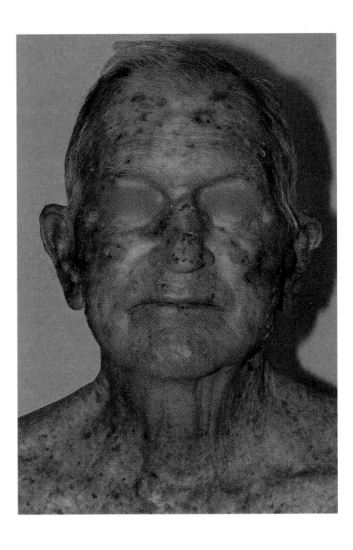

Fig. 2.8
Diagnosis: Actinic keratoses-Diffuse
Clinical Description: Diffuse, pink, scaly papules
coalescing into larger plaques on the forearms

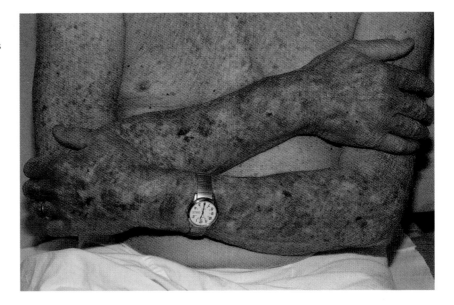

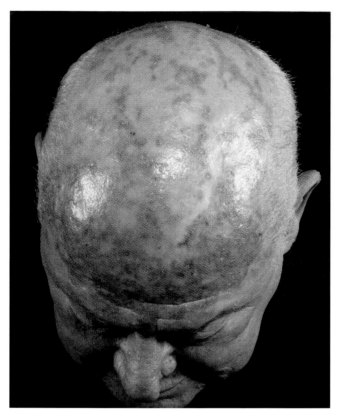

Fig. 2.9
Diagnosis: Actinic keratoses-Diffuse
Clinical Description: Diffuse, pink, scaly patches on the forehead
and scalp

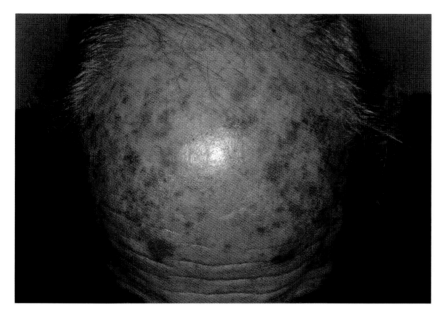

Fig. 2.10
Diagnosis: Actinic keratoses-Diffuse
Clinical Description: Diffuse, pink, scaly patches
on the forehead and frontal scalp

Fig. 2.11
Diagnosis: Actinic keratoses
Clinical Description: Pink, scaly plaque on the nasal tip

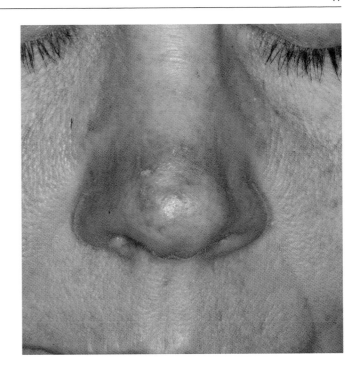

Fig. 2.12
Diagnosis: Actinic keratosis
Clinical Description: Pink, scaly plaque on left cheek

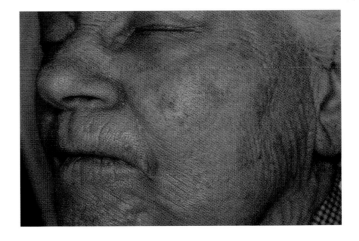

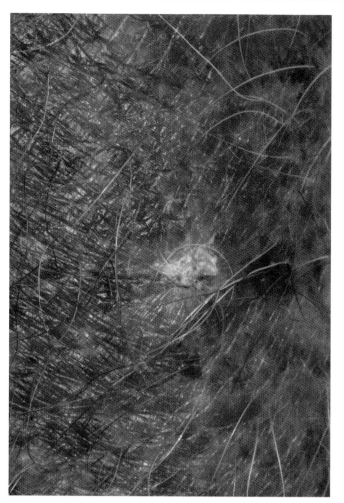

Fig. 2.13
Diagnosis: Hypertrophic Actinic Keratosis
Clinical Description: Hyperkeratotic papule

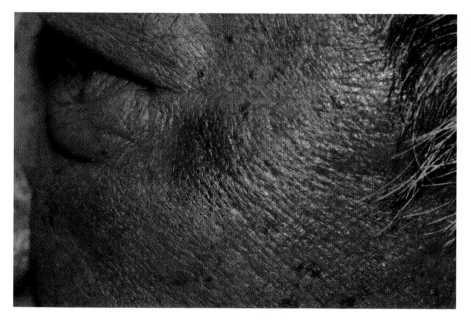

Fig. 2.14
Diagnosis: Pigmented Actinic Keratosis
Clinical Description: Hyperpigmented,
minimally elevated, keratotic plaque on
left cheek

Fig. 2.15
Diagnosis: Pigmented Actinic Keratosis
Clinical Description: Hyperpigmented, rough,
keratotic plaque

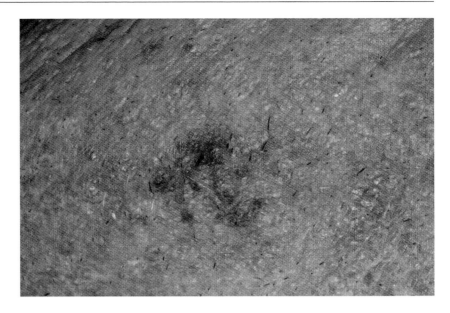

2.4 Clinical Images of Mimickers of Actinic Keratosis

Fig. 2.16
Diagnosis: Seborrheic Dermatitis-chronic and inflamed
Clinical Description: Pink patches with overlying dry scale and serous
crust along postauricular sulcus

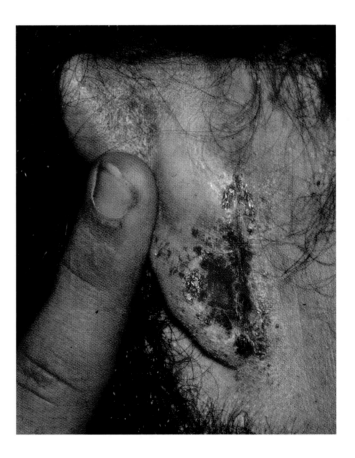

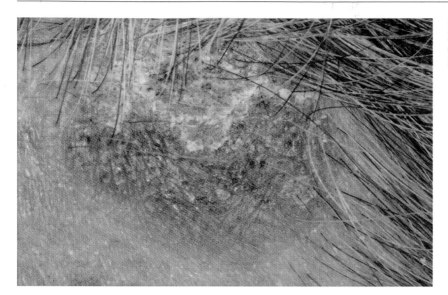

Fig. 2.17
Diagnosis: Seborrheic Dermatitis-chronic
Clinical Description: Pink, scaly plaque along
hairline with plate-like, adherent white scale

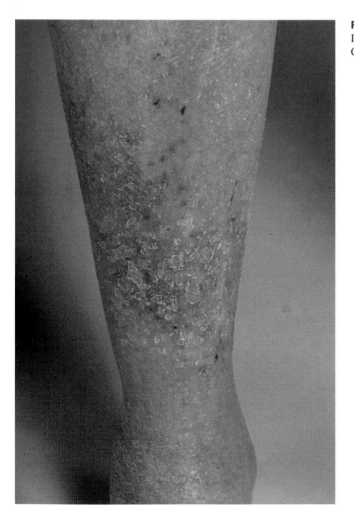

Fig. 2.18
Diagnosis: Xerosis (dry skin)
Clinical Description: Pink patch with fine white scale on lower leg

Fig. 2.19
Diagnosis: Xerosis (dry skin)
Clinical Description: erythematous nummular
plaque with fine white scale on lower leg

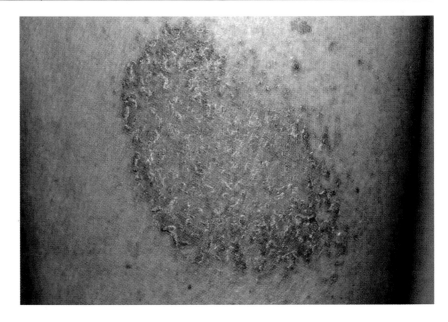

Fig. 2.20
Diagnosis: Hand eczema
Clinical Description: Pink, inflamed, scaly
patches on dorsal hand

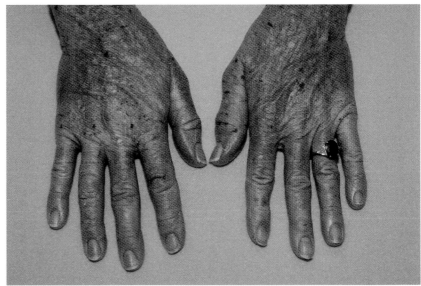

Fig. 2.21
Diagnosis: Seborrheic Keratoses-inflamed
Clinical Description: Multiple stuck-on appearing
brown papules and plaques on back. In the center
are several lesions that are pink and inflamed.
Inflamed seborrheic keratoses can be scratched
off or fall off and leave a pink scaly area that can
resemble an actinic keratosis

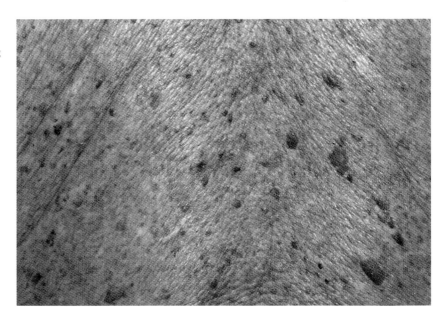

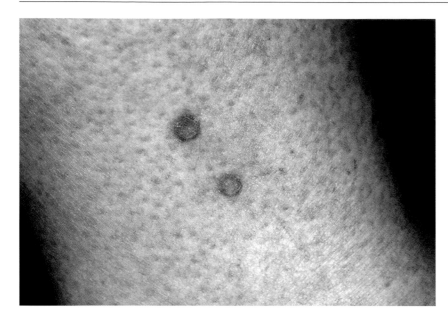

Fig. 2.22
Diagnosis: Porokeratosis
Clinical Description: Erythematous plaque with well-defined peripheral rim of scale

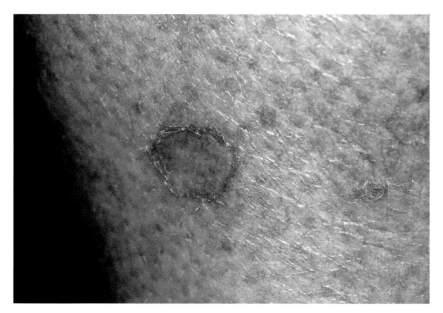

Fig. 2.23
Diagnosis: Porokeratosis
Clinical Description: Erythematous plaque with well-defined peripheral rim of scale

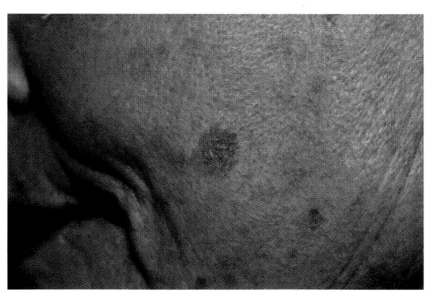

Fig. 2.24
Diagnosis: Squamous cell carcinoma in situ
Clinical Description: Pink, scaly, plaque on the left cheek

Fig. 2.25
Diagnosis: Seborrheic Dermatitis
Clinical Description: Erythema and scale around mouth and particularly within nasolabial fold

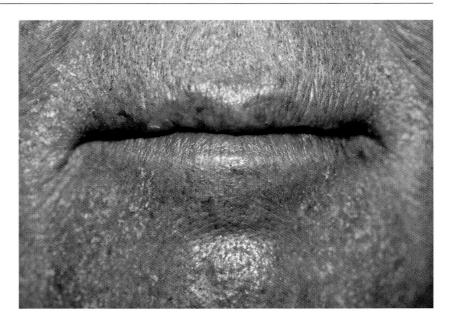

Fig. 2.26
Diagnosis: Seborrheic dermatitis
Clinical Description: Pink patches with yellow, greasy, adherent scale on face, particularly along alar groove of nose

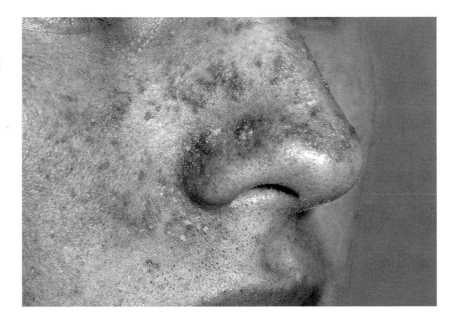

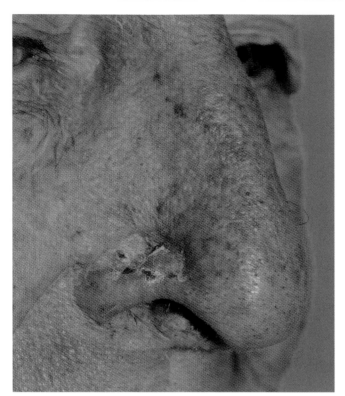

Fig. 2.27
Diagnosis: Basal Cell Carcinoma
Clinical Description: erythematous, sclerotic plaque with overlying scale on the right nasal alar crease and ala

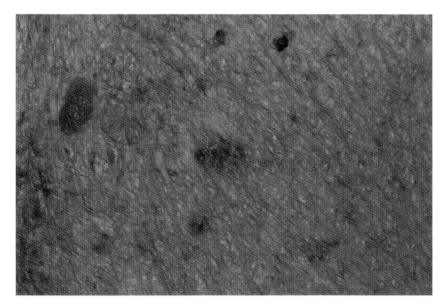

Fig. 2.28
Diagnosis: Basal Cell Carcinoma
Clinical Description: erythematous, scaly, minimally elevated plaque

Fig. 2.29
Diagnosis: Lichenoid Keratosis
Clinical Description: erythematous, scaly,
minimally elevated plaque

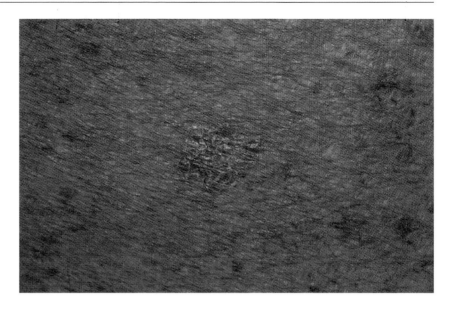

Fig. 2.30
Diagnosis: Discoid Lupus
Clinical Description: scaly, erythematous plaque with adherent
overlying scale in the conchal bowl

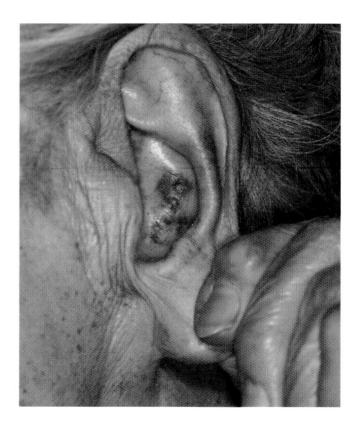

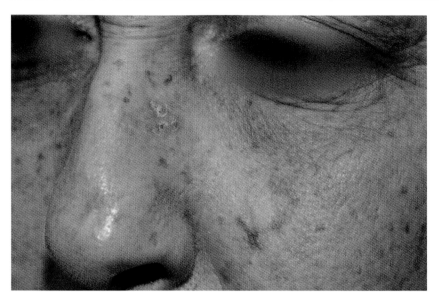

Fig. 2.31
Diagnosis: Discoid Lupus
Clinical Description: scaly, erythematous plaque
with adherent overlying scale on the left nasal
sidewall

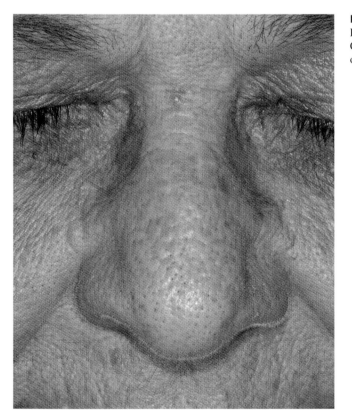

Fig. 2.32
Diagnosis: Microcystic Adnexal Carcinoma (MAC)
Clinical Description: erythematous, scaly, minimally elevated plaque
on the nasal root

Fig. 2.33
Diagnosis: Amelanotic Melanoma
Clinical Description: erythematous, scaly, minimally elevated plaque on the left alar rim

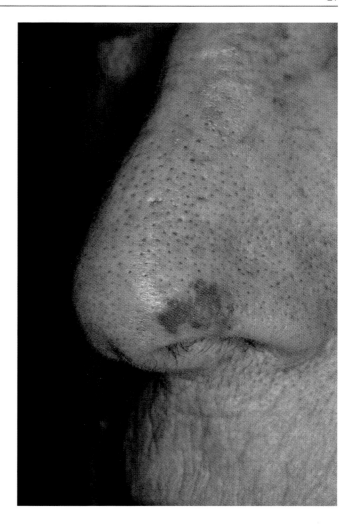

Fig. 2.34
Diagnosis: superficially invasive Squamous Cell Carcinoma
Clinical Description: erythematous, scaly, minimally elevated plaque on the right lateral brow

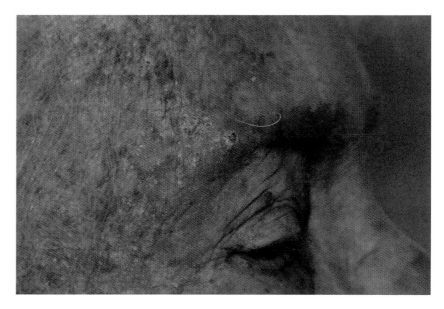

References

Ackerman AB, Mones JM (2006) Solar (actinic) keratosis is squamous cell carcinoma. Br J Dermatol 155(1):9–22

Askew DA, Mickan SM, Soyer HP et al (2009) Effectiveness of 5-fluo-rouracil treatment for actinic keratosis-a systematic review of randomized controlled trials. Int J Dermatol 48(5):453–463

Tierney E, Barker A, Ahdout J et al (2009) Photodynamic therapy for the treatment of cutaneous neoplasia, inflammatory disorders, and photoaging. Dermatol Surg 35(5):725–746

Nonmelanoma Skin Cancer

3

3.1 Introduction

Skin cancers are broadly divided into melanoma and non-melanoma skin cancers (NMSC). Due to the relatively low risk of metastasis from squamous cell carcinoma (SCC) and the extremely low risk of metastasis from basal cell carcinoma (BCC), these, the two most common cutaneous malignancies, are, for the most part, considered jointly as NMSC. This term is a bit of a misnomer; there are many other cutaneous malignancies that are not melanoma, but because of their more aggressive clinical behavior, they tend not to be grouped under this moniker.

BCC is the most common type of skin cancer. It arises from the basal keratinocytes of the epidermis. The most common presentation is a pink, pearly papule or plaque on sun-exposed skin. Risk factors for BCC include fair complexion, chronic sun exposure, and ionizing radiation. Patients older than 40 years of age are more prone to BCC, although recent data have shown that the incidence of BCC is increasing in younger patients (Christenson et al. 2005).

The most common location for BCC is the face, particularly the nose. Patient may relay a history of a bump or blemish that never heals completely or bleeds easily. As BCC tends to grow slowly, a lesion may be present for months or years before a patient seeks medical attention. For this reason, patients that are at risk should have routine complete skin examinations. Proper lighting is paramount in detecting BCC at their earliest stages.

SCC is the second most common type of skin cancer. It, too, arises from the epidermal keratinocytes. It typically presents as a scaly papule, plaque, or nodule on sun-exposed skin. Risk factors for SCC are the same as those for BCC and, in addition, include cigarette smoking. The most common location for SCC is the skin of the head and neck. Like BCC, it is more commonly seen in older patients, although younger patients with significant sun exposure and a fair complexion have an increased risk of developing SCC. Unlike BCC, SCC can grow rapidly and has an increased risk of metastasis, especially in chronically immunosuppressed patients, such as organ transplant recipients.

A. Hendi and J.C. Martinez, *Atlas of Skin Cancers*,
DOI: 10.1007/978-3-642-13399-2_3, © Mayo Foundation for Medical Education and Research 2011

3.2 Treatment of Nonmelanoma Skin Cancer

There are numerous methods of treating biopsy-proven NMSC. They vary depending on the diagnosis, histologic subtype of the cancer, anatomic location, and a variety of clinical factors. Several of the factors involved in deciding on the management of a particular lesion are listed in Table 3.1.

Recurrent and metastatic tumors account for the majority of morbidity and mortality associated with skin cancer, and tumors that show any of the factors associated with recurrence and metastases should be considered "high risk." In particular, certain histologic subtypes of BCC and SCC are associated with higher recurrence rates. Tumors showing none of these factors can be considered "low-risk." These risk factors are listed in Table 3.2. This determination is critical in the management of skin cancers, both in determining the method of treatment and in determining which physician should treat the lesion.

Figures 3.1 and 3.2 can be used to help decide what treatments may be most appropriate in the management of biopsy-proven BCC and SCC.

Below, we briefly review the most commonly used methods of treatment of skin cancer. Table 3.3 lists some advantages and disadvantages of each.

3.2.1 Topical Treatments

As noted in Chap. 2, topical therapies, including PDT, 5-fluorouracil, and imiquimod have recently begun to be employed in the management of premalignant lesions and superficial malignancies such as superficial BCC and squamous cell

Table 3.1 Variables crucial to proper management of patients with skin cancer. (Modified and reprinted from Mayo Clinic Proceedings. With permission)

Disease factors	Patient factors	Treatment factors
Type of skin cancer	Life expectancy	Physician's skill and training
Pathologic growth pattern	Comorbid conditions	Cure rate of treatment modality
Primary vs recurrent tumor	Cosmetic concerns	Preservation of normal function
Size of tumor		Morbidity
Anatomic location		Cosmesis Cost

Table 3.2 NCCN guidelines: risk factors for recurrence of NMSC. (Modified and reprinted from Mayo Clinic Proceedings. With permission)

Clinical risk factors	Low risk	High risk
Location/size	L – <20 mm M – <10 mm H – <6 mm	L – ≥20 mm M – ≥10 mm H – ≥6 mm
Borders	Well defined	Poorly defined
Primary vs recurrent	Primary	Recurrent
Immunosuppressed patient	No	Yes
Tumor at site of prior XRT or chronic inflammatory process	No	Yes
Rapidly growing tumor[a]	No	Yes
Neurologic symptoms: pain, paresthesia, paralysis	No	Yes
Pathologic risk factors		
Subtype[b]	Nodular, superficial	Infiltrative, micronodular, sclerotic, or morpheaform
Degree of differentiation[a]	Well differentiated	Moderately or poorly differentiated
Depth: Clark's level or thickness[a]	I, II, III or <6 mm	IV, V, or ≥6 mm
Perineural or vascular involvement	No	Yes

L areas at low risk for recurrence: trunk, extremities, *M* areas at middle risk for recurrence: cheeks, forehead, neck, scalp, *H* areas at high risk for recurrence: central face, eyelids, nose, chin, mandible, preauricular and postauricular skin/sulci, temple, ear, genitalia, hands, and feet
[a]Applicable only to SCC
[b]Applicable only to BCC

carcinoma in situ. The data regarding use of PDT for superficial BCC and SCC in situ are relatively limited, though some treatment protocols have resulted in promising cure rates (Tierney et al. 2009).

Following some success in the treatment of actinic keratoses, imiquimod and 5-FU have been more recently approved by the FDA for the treatment of superficial BCC on the trunk and extremities. Cure rates for both of these topical treatments range from 50% to 90% depending on type of tumor, frequency of application, and duration of treatment course (Marks et al. 2004; Gross et al. 2007; Peris et al. 2005; Gollnick et al. 2008).

It is important to note that neither of these topical treatments is FDA-approved for any other histological subtype of BCC. Similarly, neither of these creams is FDA-approved for any BCC, regardless of subtype, on the skin of the face, neck, or scalp. Patient and tumor selection are critical.

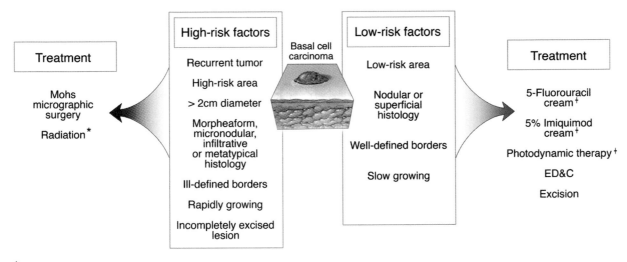

* - *Primarily considered in patients unwilling or unable to undergo surgical treatment*

† - *Primarily considered for superficial BCC on trunk/extremities*

Fig. 3.1
Treatment algorithm for BCC based on clinical and pathologic factors (modified and reprinted with permission from Mayo Clinic Proceedings)

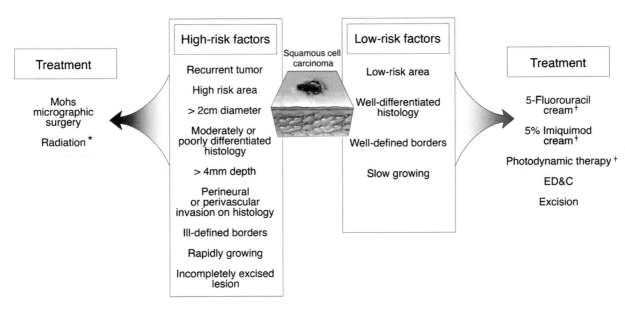

* - *Primarily considered in patients unwilling or unable to undergo surgical treatment*

† - *only considered for SCC in situ*

Fig. 3.2
Treatment algorithm for SCC based on clinical and pathologic factors (modified and reprinted with permission from Mayo Clinic Proceedings)

Table 3.3 Characteristics of common treatment methods for skin cancer. (Modified and reprinted from Mayo Clinic Proceedings. With permission)

Treatment modality	Advantages	Disadvantages
Topical creams (5-Fluorouracil/Imiquimod)	Simple to use Can be done by patient at home Noninvasive Potential for excellent cosmetic results May help avoid surgery	Not much long-term data regarding cure rates No margin control Only FDA-approved for a small subset of superficial skin cancers Lengthy duration of treatment course (6–16 weeks) Can lead to significant redness and irritation May "bury" persistent tumor, requiring more extensive surgical treatment in the future
PDT	Simple to perform Noninvasive technique Excellent cosmetic results feasible Minimal restriction of postprocedural activity	Specialized equipment needed No histological margin control Can be moderately painful Still investigational for treatment of skin cancer Patient must stay out of sunlight for 24–48 h
ED&C	Minimal equipment needed Simple to perform Inexpensive Little to no restriction of postoperative activity	No histological margin control Slower healing by second intention Greater potential for suboptimal cosmesis
Mohs surgery	100% microscopically controlled margins Highest conservation of normal tissue and structures Highest cure rates Best cosmetic results of surgical options	Specialized training and facilities needed Increased time for complete margin control Postoperative activity restriction if reconstructed
Excision	Relatively easy to perform Some margin control (more than ED&C) More rapid healing with primary repair Good cosmetic results	Subtotal margin control (less than Mohs surgery) Requires equipment and assistance Lack of tissue conservation Postoperative activity restriction if reconstructed
XRT	Good cure rates for primary and recurrent cancers Helpful in inoperable cases or patients unsuitable for surgery	No histologic margin control Most expensive Repetitious treatments over 2–6 weeks Potential for carcinogenesis in young patients

3.2.2 Electrodesiccation and Curettage (ED&C)

This is a simple way of treating skin cancers in the office. This technique is most effective for the destruction of well-defined, superficial skin cancers (e.g., superficial BCC or SCC in situ). Cure rates for well-demarcated, primary superficial skin cancers can exceed 80% (Rodriguez-Vigil et al. 2007) (Figs. 3.3–3.15).

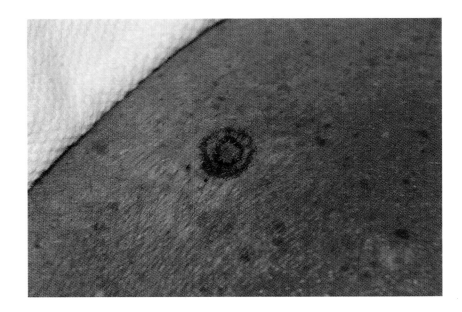

Fig. 3.3
Lesion or biopsy site is identified, cleaned, and appropriate margins are delineated

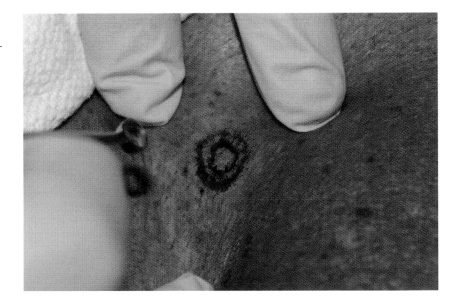

Fig. 3.4
After anesthetic has been infiltrated, three-point traction is applied using two fingers of nondominant hand and fifth finger of dominant hand. A 4-mm curette is held with pencil grip

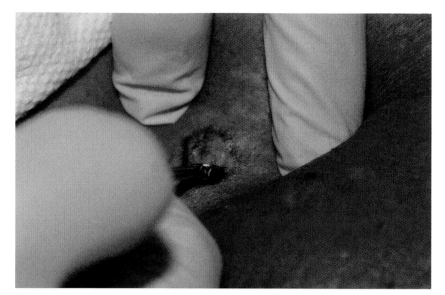

Fig. 3.5
While keeping three-point traction, the curette is used to firmly debride the lesion, scraping off epithelium and any friable tissue at the base and periphery

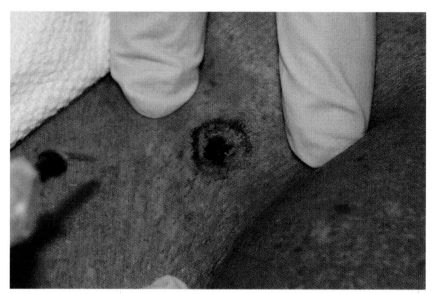

Fig. 3.6
Appearance of the wound after a single "pass" with curette

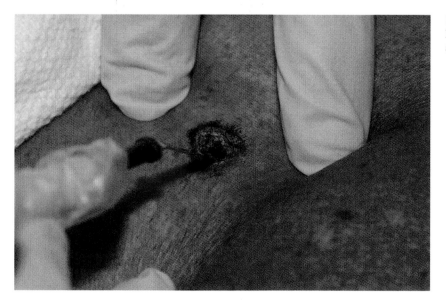

Fig. 3.7
Electrodesiccation is used to treat the periphery and the entire base of the curetted area

Fig. 3.8
Appearance of the wound after a single pass with
curettage and electrodesiccation

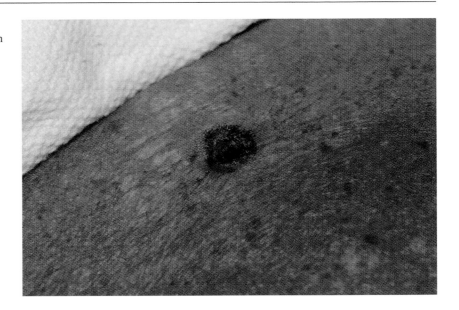

Fig. 3.9
Curettage is repeated as in Fig 3.5, taking care to
remove all the char at the periphery and base of
the wound

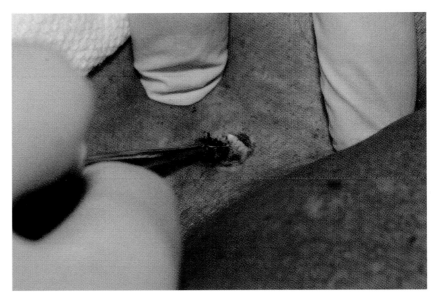

Fig. 3.10
Appearance of the wound after second pass with
curette

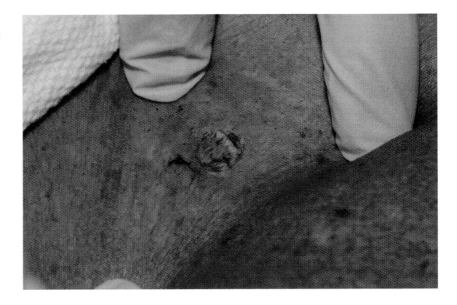

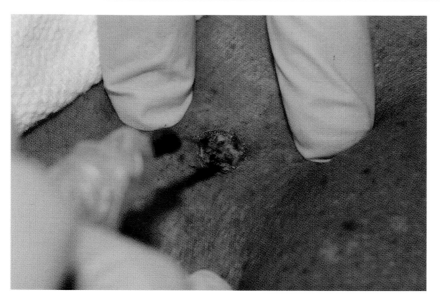

Fig. 3.11
Electrodesiccation is repeated, taking care to completely to completely treat the periphery first

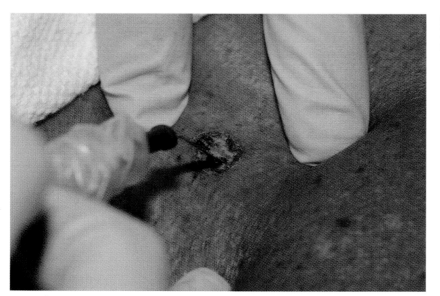

Fig. 3.12
Electrodesiccation then used to "fill in" the remainder of defect after periphery is treated

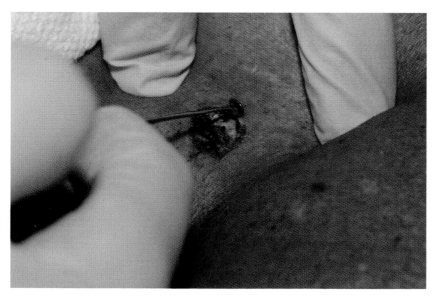

Fig. 3.13
A 2-mm curette is used for third and final pass of curettage, again taking care to remove all char

Fig. 3.14
Appearance of wound after third pass with curette

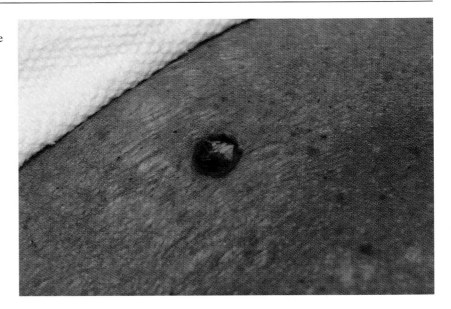

Fig. 3.15
Appearance of wound after third and final pass
with electrodesiccation. Note contraction of
tissue from electrosurgical treatment. Further
contraction as wound heals will result in a
hypopigmented scar significantly smaller than
the originally marked area

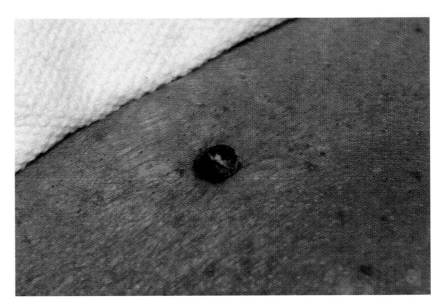

3.2.3 Excision

Surgical excision with margins of clinically uninvolved skin is the mainstay of treatment for NMSC on the trunk and extremities. The majority of these excisions are performed using a standard elliptical excision and primary closure. BCC and SCC with low-risk characteristics are excised, if feasible, with 4 mm margins; 6 mm margins should be used for high-risk BCC and SCC if surgical excision is desired and Mohs surgery is not available or feasible. (Brodland and Zitelli 1992; Wolf and Zitelli 1987). Systematic reviews using actuarial data report 5-year cure rates of 90–92% following standard surgical excision (Rowe et al. 1992, 1989) (Figs. 3.16–3.40).

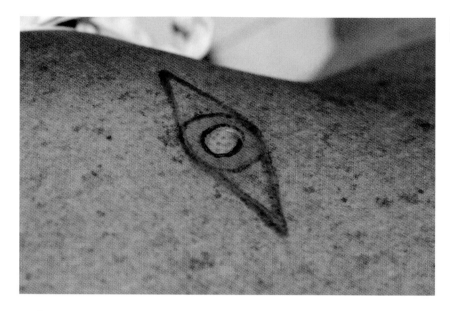

Fig. 3.16
Biopsy site and margins marked. Ellipse planned

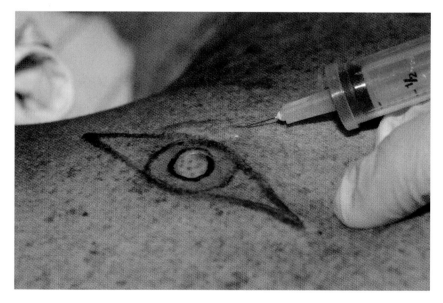

Fig. 3.17
Needle is inserted into the dermis and anesthetic is injected. Note the wheal

Fig. 3.18
Needle advanced while infiltrating anesthetic

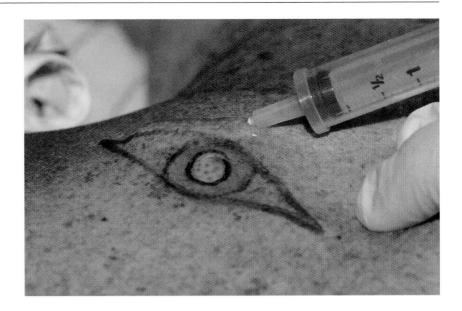

Fig. 3.19
Fanning technique: needle is redirected without completely withdrawing from the skin

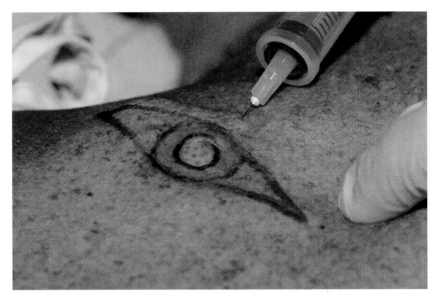

Fig. 3.20
Needle is advanced to anesthetize the center and depth of the ellipse

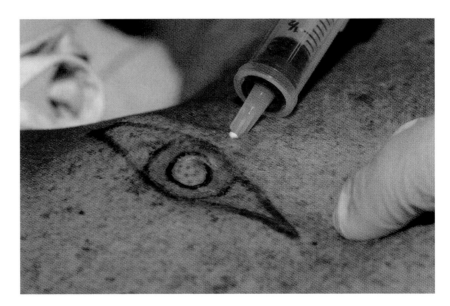

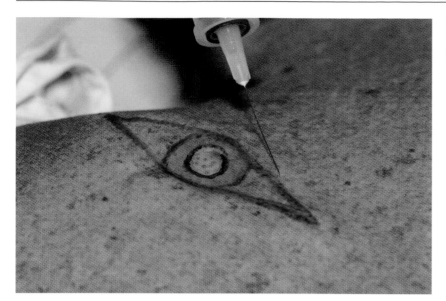

Fig. 3.21
Testing for anesthesia by gently touching with needle tip around the periphery of the ellipse

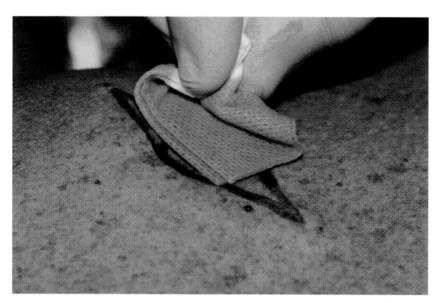

Fig. 3.22
Surgical site is prepped

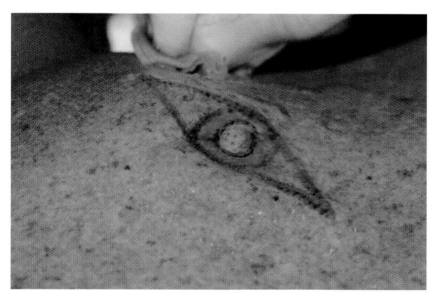

Fig. 3.23
Overlapping, concentric circles moving away from the planned ellipse

Fig. 3.24
Incision is started, keeping the blade edge
perpendicular to the skin. The blade is rocked
back so that the belly, not the tip, of the blade
is in contact with the skin surface

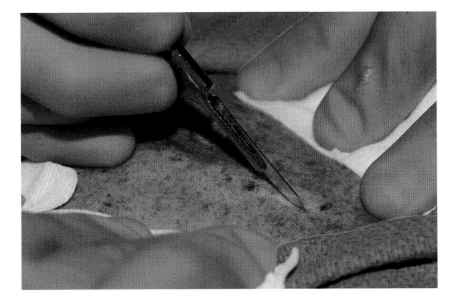

Fig. 3.25
Firm pressure is used to incise at once through
the dermis and into the subcutaneous fat

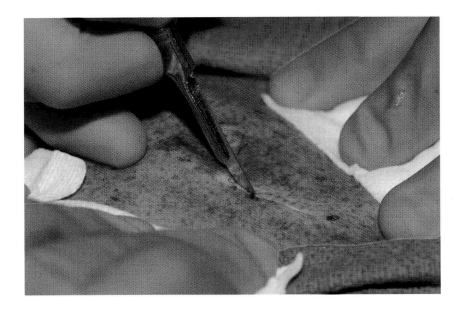

Fig. 3.26
Care is taken to keep the blade edge
perpendicular to the skin surface

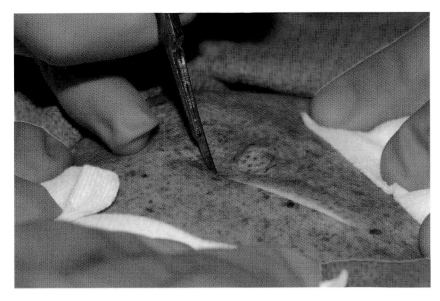

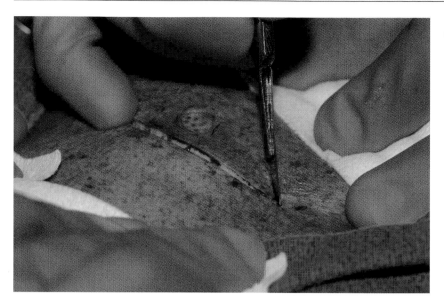

Fig. 3.27
The opposite edge in similarly incised

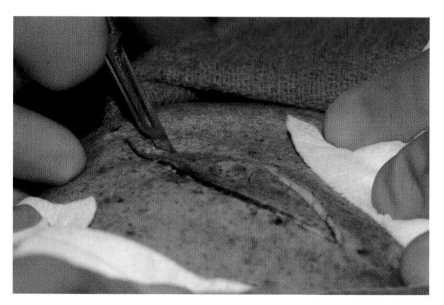

Fig. 3.28
Care is taken when incising near the apices not
to leave hash marks in the skin edge

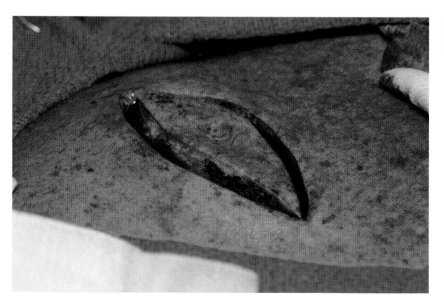

Fig. 3.29
The specimen "floats" when completely freed
from dermal edges

Fig. 3.30
(**a**, **b**) The blade is used to remove specimen at a single, planar depth within the subcutaneous tissue

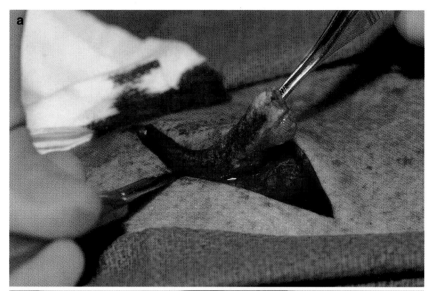

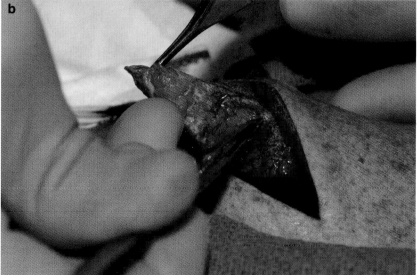

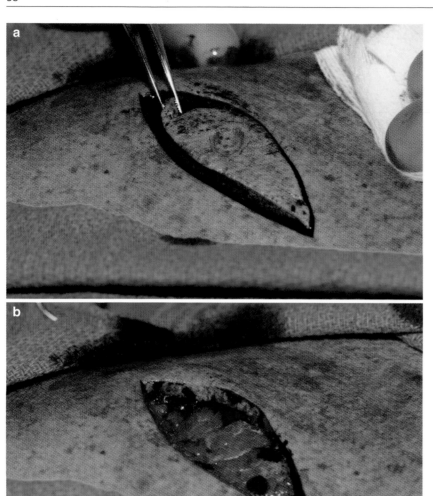

Fig. 3.31
(**a**, **b**) The defect is now ready to be prepared for closure

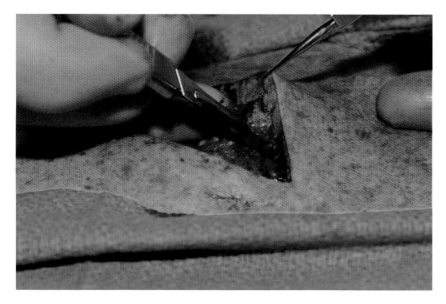

Fig. 3.32
Preparing to undermine using sharp dissection. Start at either apex

Fig. 3.33
Skin hooks are used to provide gentle traction. Continue undermining along the entire periphery of the wound edge. Be sure to fully undermine apices of the ellipse

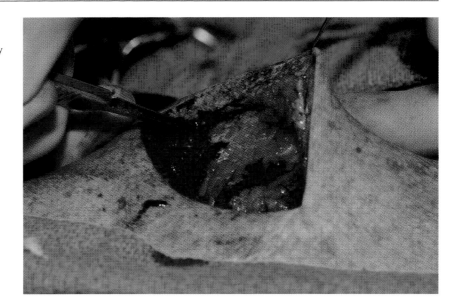

Fig. 3.34
Pinpoint electrodesiccation is used to obtain hemostasis

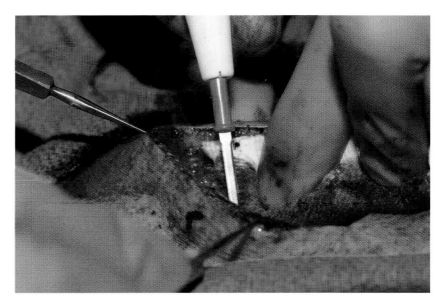

Fig. 3.35
A deep plication suture is placed to reduce wound closure tension

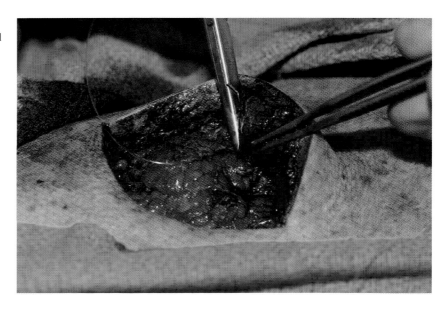

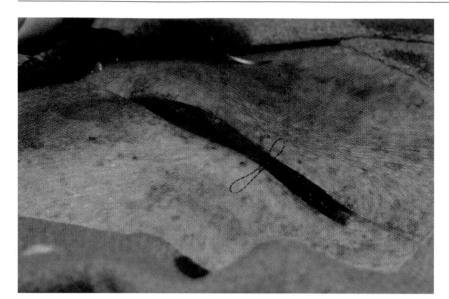

Fig. 3.36
Plication suture in place

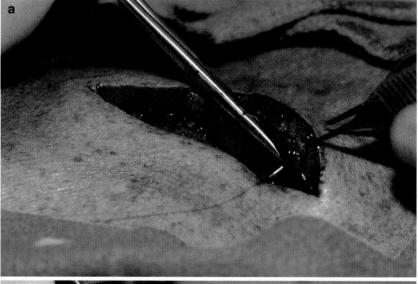

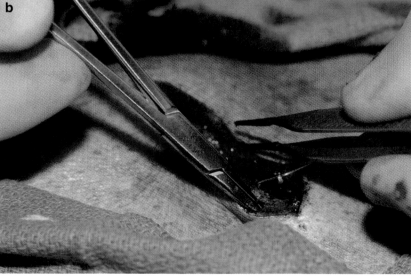

Fig. 3.37
(**a**–**c**) The first buried vertical mattress suture is placed

Fig. 3.37
(continued)

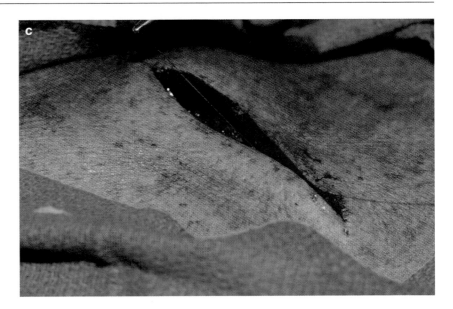

Fig. 3.38
Four buried mattress sutures in place. Note good eversion and complete apposition of dermal and epidermal edges

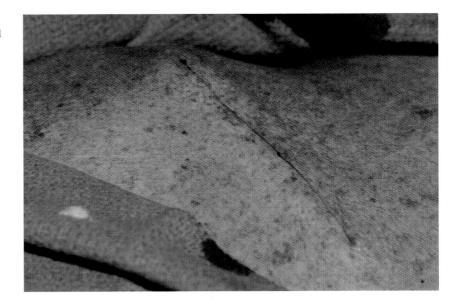

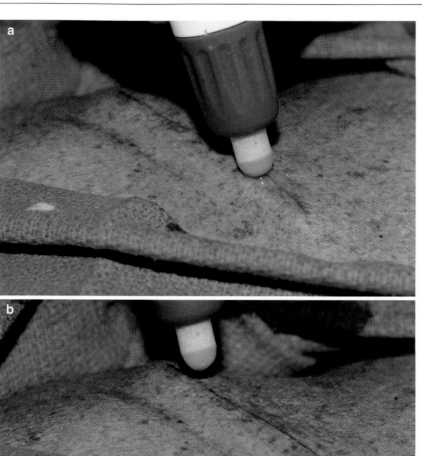

Fig. 3.39
(**a**, **b**) Skin glue is applied along the length of
the incision to seal epidermal edges

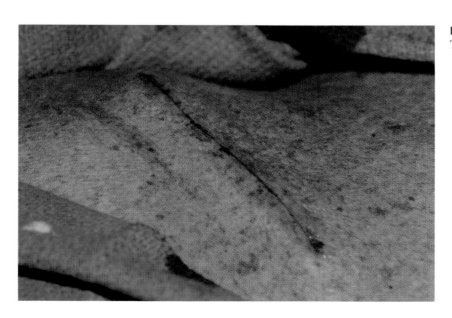

Fig. 3.40
The surgical site is now ready for a bandage

3.2.4 Mohs Micrographic Surgery

Mohs micrographic surgery is a specialized technique of excision and margin examination that provides the highest cure rates and maximum conservation of normal tissue. The cure rates associated with Mohs surgery for the treatment of BCC and SCC are well established and approach 99%. The technique is particularly well suited for high-risk tumors such as those with aggressive histologic patterns (infiltrative or sclerosing BCC, spindle cell SCC), recurrent tumors, larger lesions (>2 cm on the body, greater than 0.6–1.0 cm on the face), or areas where tissue conservation is of great importance (e.g., eyelids, nose, ears, lips, genitalia, and shins).

The method is performed in stages, whereby the surgeon initially anesthetizes and excises the clinically evident tumor or biopsy site. While the patient waits with a bandage in place, the surgeon examines 100% of the surgical margin to ensure that the entire tumor has been removed. If the tumor is completely excised in the first stage, the patient is deemed "clear" of tumor, and the defect is ready to be repaired. If, however, there is residual tumor noted on the examined tissue, the surgeon is able to precisely delineate what tissue is still involved and, after marking it on an anatomic map, return to the patient for a second stage of tissue removal. The process is repeated until there is no further evidence of malignancy.

The Mohs technique ensures both that 100% of the surgical margin is histologically examined and that *only* the malignant tissue – with a minimal margin of normal tissue – is removed. This stands in marked contrast to the less than 1% margin examination that occurs with traditional "bread-loafed" specimens from standard excisions. Once the malignancy has been completely extirpated, the tumor-free defect is ready for immediate reconstruction. The majority of Mohs surgeons repair the defect immediately, although multidisciplinary collaboration with plastic surgeons, facial plastic surgeons, and oculoplastic surgeons is not at all uncommon.

It is the authors' opinion that this technique should be practiced only by fellowship-trained individuals, who have done an additional 1–2 years of training to acquire expertise in the fields of cutaneous oncology, histopathologic interpretation of frozen sections, and reconstruction of soft tissue defects (Figs. 3.41–3.52).

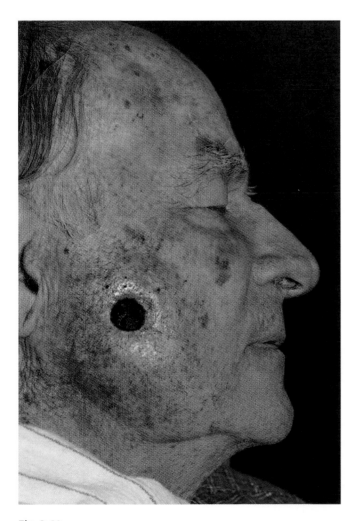

Fig. 3.41
Biopsy site of primary ulcerated BCC on the right cheek

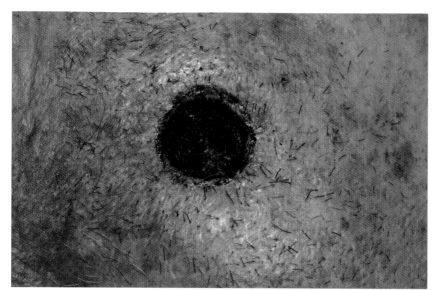

Fig. 3.42
The clinical edge of tumor is delineated along with a 1–2-mm margin of normal-appearing skin

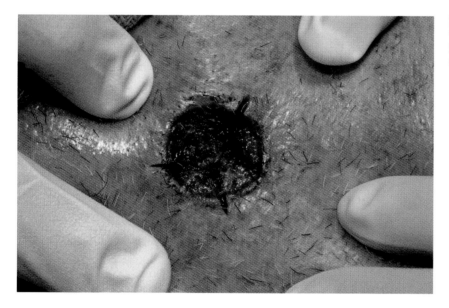

Fig. 3.43
The edge of the defect is nicked with scoring incisions to help maintain orientation of tissue once it is removed

Fig. 3.44
(**a–c**) The entire periphery is incised

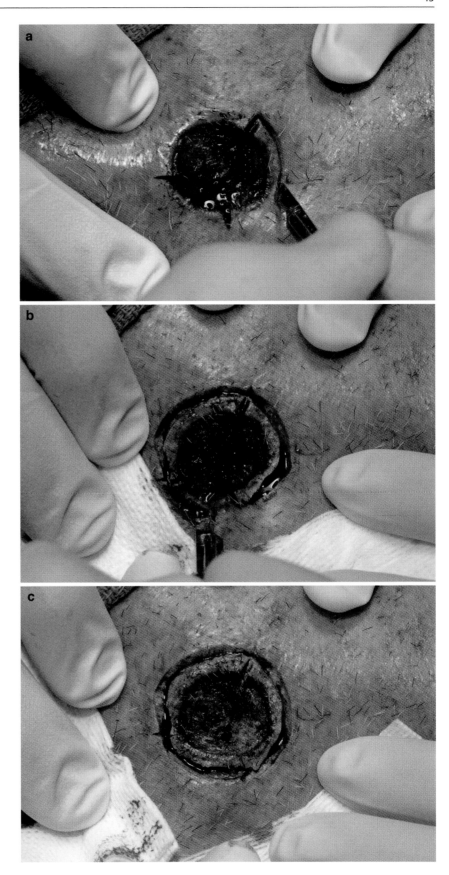

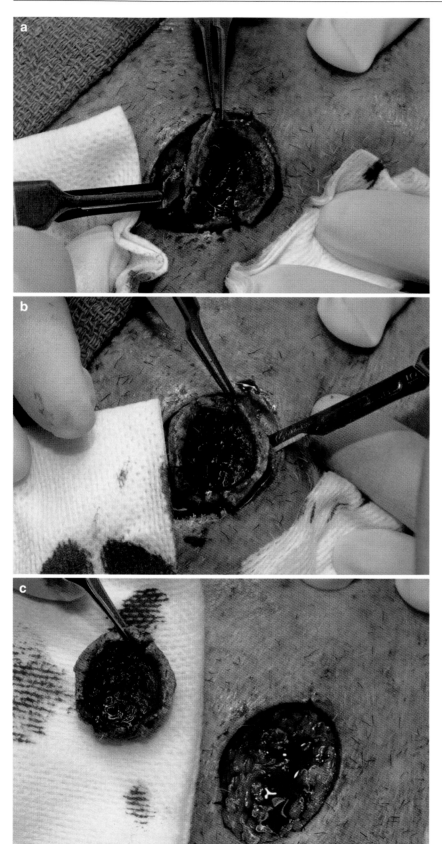

Fig. 3.45
(**a–c**) The specimen is completely excised, and special care is taken to maintain in vivo orientation

Fig. 3.46
The specimen is transferred from the patient directly onto an illustrated card to maintain orientation. The tissue is then divided along the original scoring incisions; in this case the specimen is trisected. The tissue is then inked, and a corresponding color-coded map is drawn

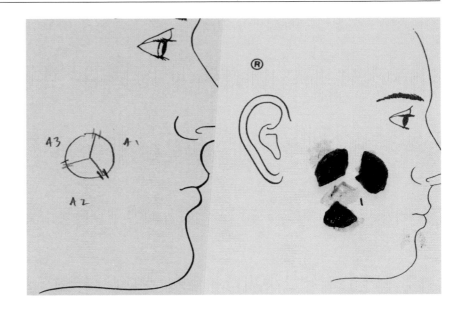

Fig. 3.47
Frozen sectioning is performed, and glass slides are produced. Each section includes the entire depth and peripheral edge of the block of tissue from which it was cut. Careful histologic examination is performed by the Mohs surgeon, and the areas of positivity are marked on the tissue map. In this instance the majority of the peripheral edge of section A1 is positive for malignancy. This is marked with red pencil on the Mohs map. The remaining peripheral edges and entire base of the defect are already clear of malignancy at this point

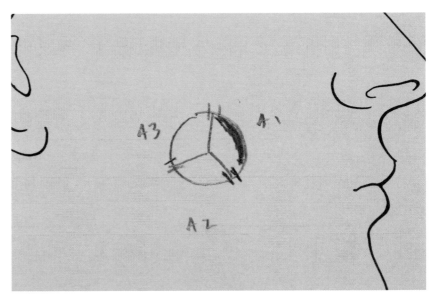

Fig. 3.48
For illustrative purposes, the initial scoring incisions, as well as the area of positivity, are delineated on the patient's skin with a surgical marking pen

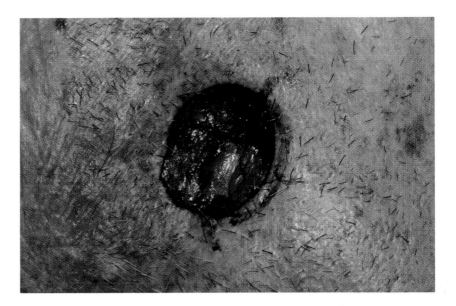

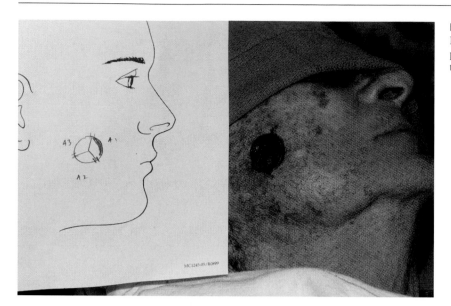

Fig. 3.49
Here, one can appreciate that the area of
positivity marked on the patient corresponds
to the area noted on microscopic evaluation

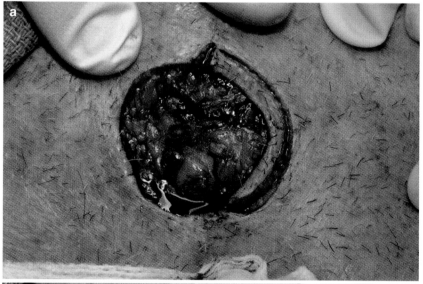

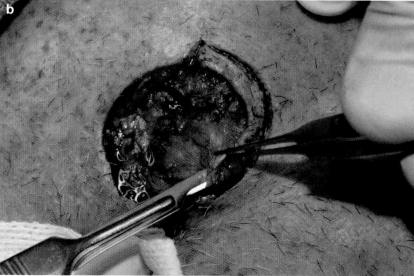

Fig. 3.50
(**a**, **b**) The second stage of Mohs surgery is
performed, removing only the area noted to
be involved by residual tumor

Fig. 3.51
As with the first stage, this second layer of tissue is inked and mapped

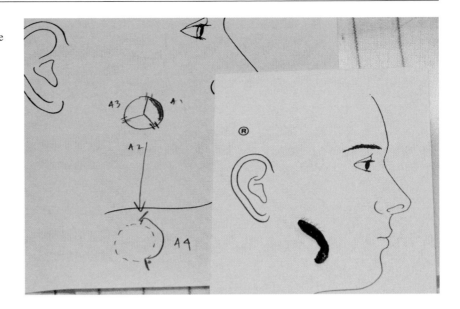

Fig. 3.52
The second layer was noted to be clear of malignancy. The postoperative, tumor-free defect is shown here, ready for reconstruction

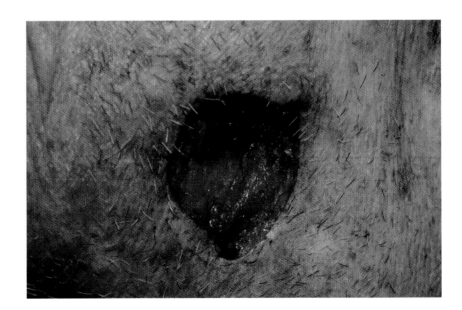

3.2.5 Radiotherapy

Radiotherapy can be quite effective in the primary treatment of nonmelanoma skin cancer, with cure rates of over 90% in properly selected patients and tumors (Voss and Kim-Sing 1998). Because there is no margin examination performed and the cure rates are relatively lower than those seen with surgical treatments, radiotherapy is usually reserved for patients who are either unable or unwilling to undergo surgical treatment. It is also indicated for treatment of tumors that are deemed inoperable or whose complete surgical removal will result in significant disfigurement or extensive reconstructive efforts.

3.3 Clinical Images of BCC (Figs. 3.53–3.75)

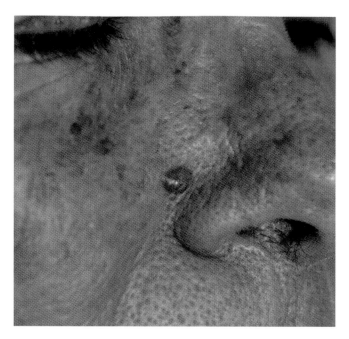

Fig. 3.53
Diagnosis: BCC-nodular
Clinical Description: Pink, pearly, telangiectatic, dome-shaped papule on the right nasofacial sulcus

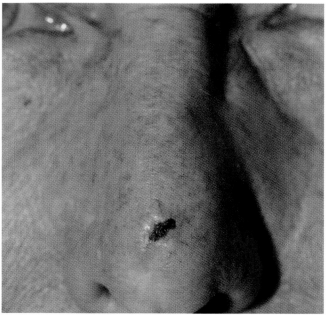

Fig. 3.55
Diagnosis: BCC
Clinical Description: Pink, pearly, eroded, telangiectatic plaque on the nasal tip

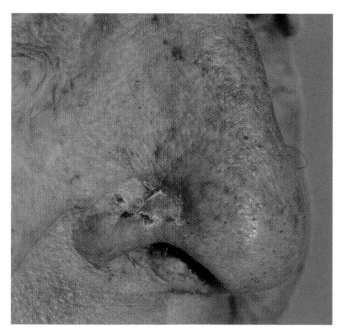

Fig. 3.54
Diagnosis: BCC-infiltrative
Clinical Description: Pinkly sclerotic, ill-defined plaque with contraction of the right alar rim

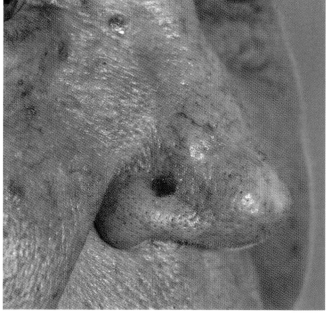

Fig. 3.56
Diagnosis: BCC
Clinical Description: Pink, pearly, eroded plaque on the right alar groove

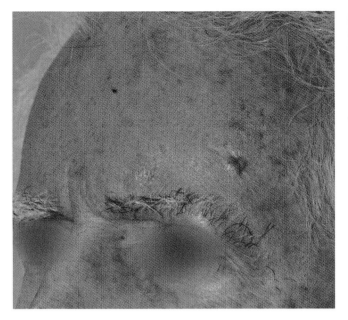

Fig. 3.57
Diagnosis: BCC
Clinical Description: Pink, pearly, plaque on left forehead

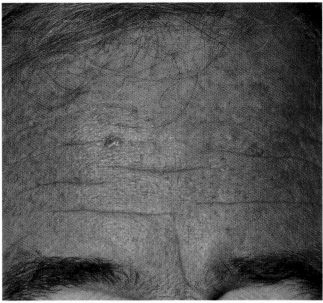

Fig. 3.58
Diagnosis: BCC
Clinical Description: Pink, pearly papule on right forehead

Fig. 3.59
Diagnosis: BCC-micronodular
Clinical Description: Depressed, sclerotic,
ill-defined, pearly plaque on left upper forehead

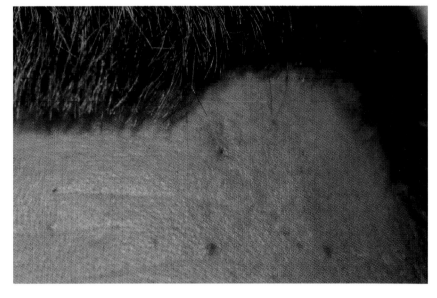

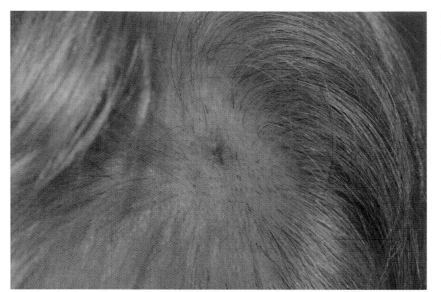

Fig. 3.60
Diagnosis: BCC
Clinical Description: Pink, eroded, pearly, plaque
on the scalp

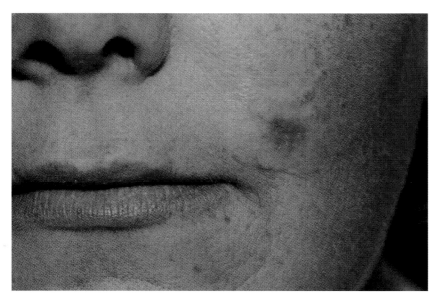

Fig. 3.61
Diagnosis: BCC-morpheaform
Clinical Description: Pink, depressed, ill-defined
plaque surrounding sclerotic-appearing hypopigmented skin on the left cheek

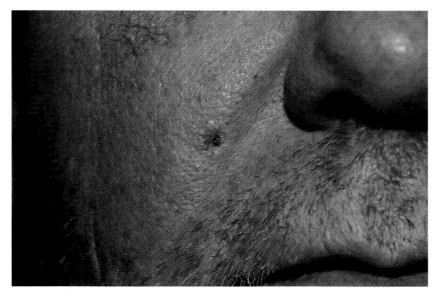

Fig. 3.62
Diagnosis: BCC
Clinical Description: Pink, ulcerated, telangiectatic plaque with rolled borders on right medial
cheek

Fig. 3.63
Diagnosis: BCC
Clinical Description: Pink, ill-defined eroded
plaque on left medial cheek

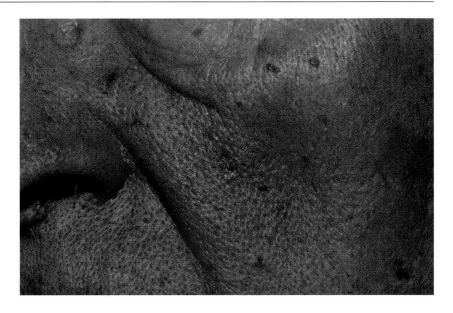

Fig. 3.64
Diagnosis: BCC
Clinical Description: Pink, pearly, plaque with
rolled borders on right upper cutaneous lip

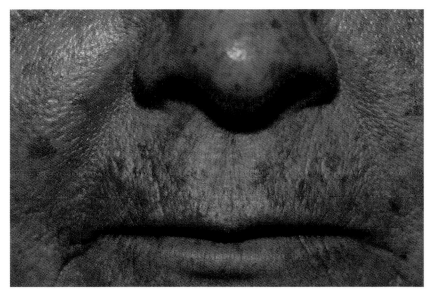

Fig. 3.65
Diagnosis: BCC-infiltrative
Clinical Description: Sclerotic, pearly, ill-defined
plaque on left upper vermilion and cutaneous lip

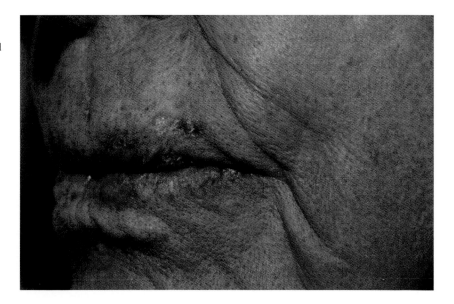

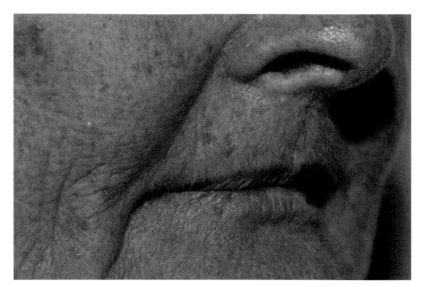

Fig. 3.66
Diagnosis: BCC-morpheaform
Clinical Description: Pink ill-defined, slightly
hypopigmented plaque on the right upper
cutaneous lip

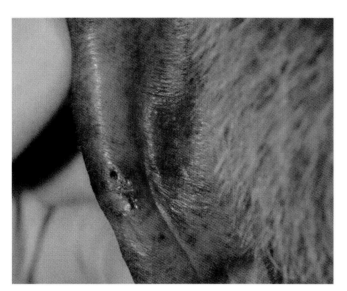

Fig. 3.67
Diagnosis: BCC-pigmented
Clinical Description: Hyperpigmented, pearly, eroded plaque
on left posterior helical rim

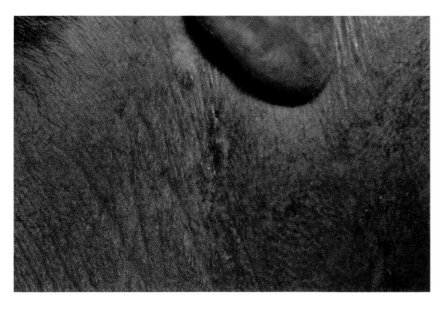

Fig. 3.68
Diagnosis: BCC
Clinical Description: Linear, ill-defined,
pink, pearly, telangiectatic plaque on right
infra-auricular neck

Fig. 3.69
Diagnosis: BCC-nodular
Clinical Description: Pink pearly, telangiectatic papule on right lateral lower eyelid

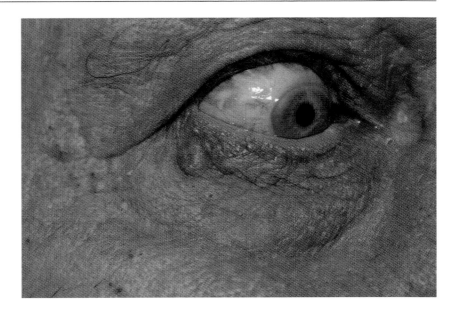

Fig. 3.70
Diagnosis: BCC-sclerotic
Clinical Description: Pink, pearly, telangiectatic plaque on left medial lower lid margin with loss of eyelashes (madarosis)

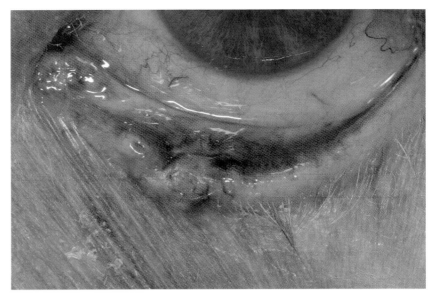

Fig. 3.71
Diagnosis: BCC-nodular
Clinical Description: Pink, pearly papule just below the right medial canthus

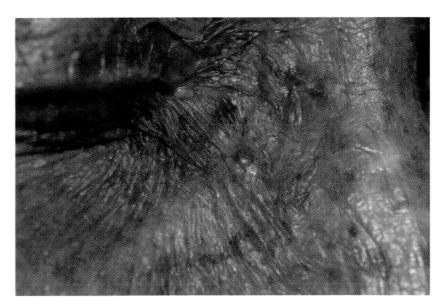

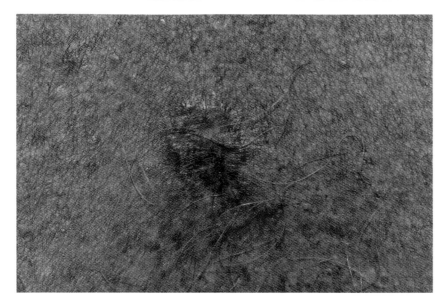

Fig. 3.72
Diagnosis: BCC
Clinical Description: Pink, ill-defined, pearly, telangiectatic plaque with rolled borders on chest

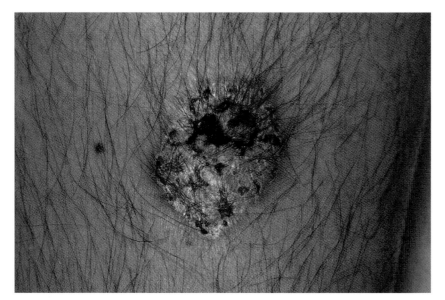

Fig. 3.73
Diagnosis: BCC
Clinical Description: Pink, scaly, eroded plaque with overlying crust on a lower leg

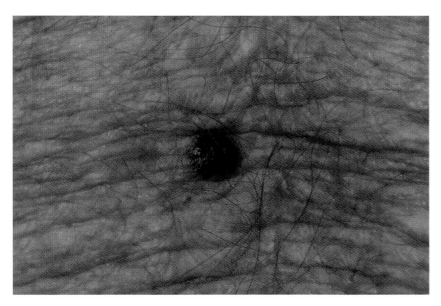

Fig. 3.74
Diagnosis: BCC-pigmented
Clinical Description: Brown, pearly, pigmented papule with pink borders on the upper extremity

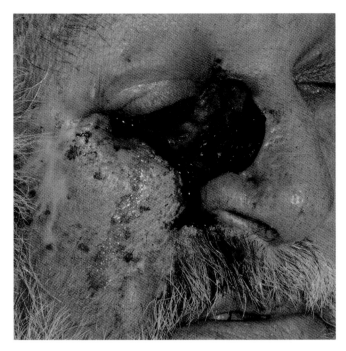

Fig. 3.75
Diagnosis: BCC-infiltrated, chronic (>20 years)
Clinical Description: Deep ulceration of the right nose, medial cheek, and lower eye lid

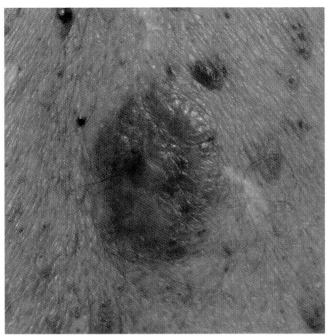

Fig. 3.77
Diagnosis: Amelonotic melanoma-invasive
Clinical Description: Pink, pearly plaque with minimal tan-brown pigment on the trunk

3.4 Clinical Images of Mimickers of BCC (Figs. 3.76–3.100)

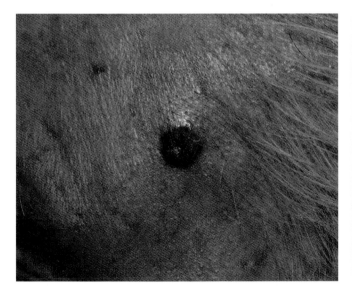

Fig. 3.76
Diagnosis: SCC
Clinical Description: Erythematous well-defined nodule on left temple

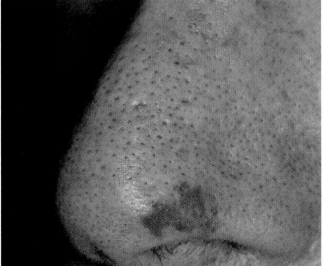

Fig. 3.78
Diagnosis: Amelonotic melanoma-superficial
Clinical Description: erythematous, rough minimally elevated plaque with peripheral pigmentation on left nasal alar rim

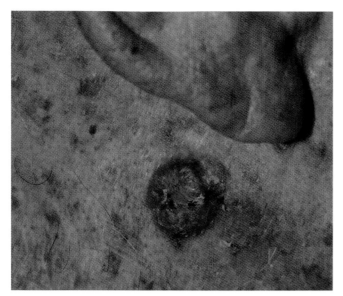

Fig. 3.79
Diagnosis: Atypical fibroxanthoma (AFX)
Clinical Description: Pink, dome-shaped scaly nodule below right ear

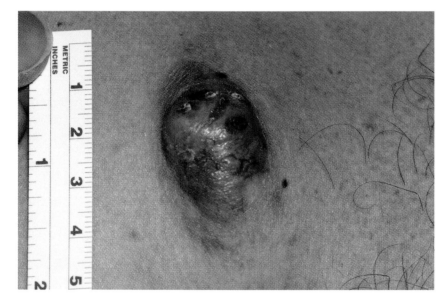

Fig. 3.80
Diagnosis: Dermatofibrosarcoma protuberans (DFSP)
Clinical Description: Purple, dome-shaped firm exophytic nodule on shoulder

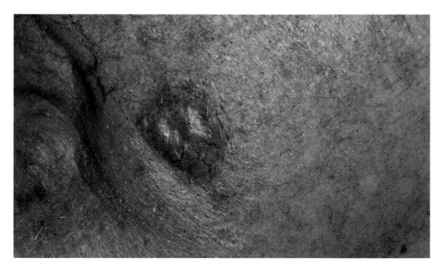

Fig. 3.81
Diagnosis: Merkel cell carcinoma (MCC)
Clinical Description: Pink, pearly, telangiectatic plaque on left medial cheek

Fig. 3.82
Diagnosis: Merkel cell carcinoma (MCC)
Clinical Description: Pink, nodule on right forearm

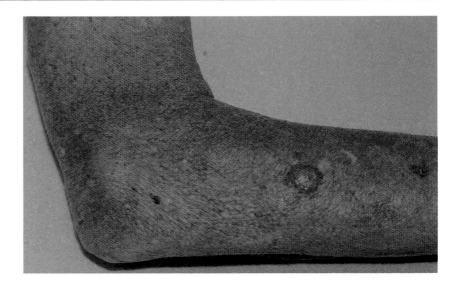

Fig. 3.83
Diagnosis: Cutaneous lymphoma
Clinical Description: Multilobular, pink, pearly plaque on mid forehead

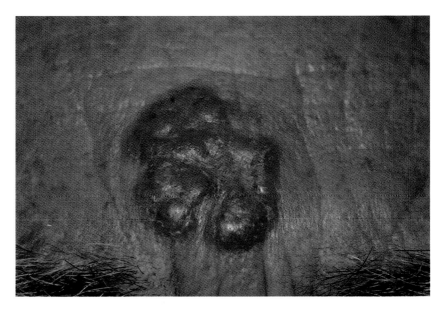

Fig. 3.84
Diagnosis: Molluscum contagiosum
Clinical Description: Pink, dome-shaped papule

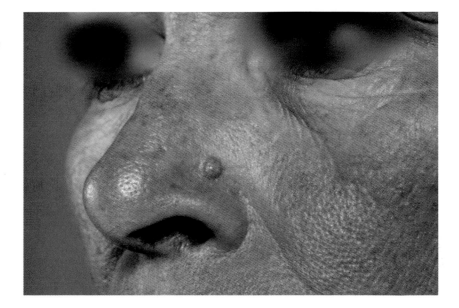

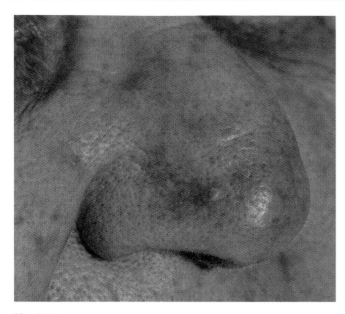

Fig. 3.85
Diagnosis: Sebaceous hyperplasia
Clinical Description: Yellowish, telangiectatic papule with central depression on the right lateral nasal tip

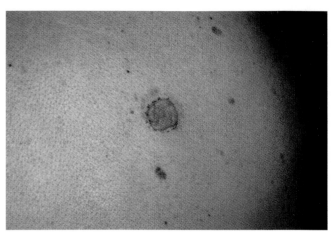

Fig. 3.88
Diagnosis: Neurofibroma
Clinical Description: Soft, compressible, pink, papule located on the trunk

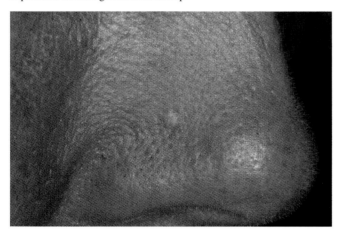

Fig. 3.86
Diagnosis: Fibrous papule
Clinical Description: Pink, opaque papule on right alar crease

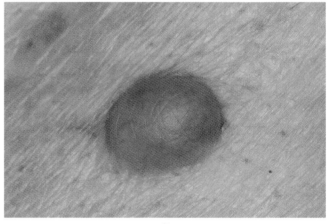

Fig. 3.89
Diagnosis: Neurofibroma
Clinical Description: Soft, compressible, pink, papule

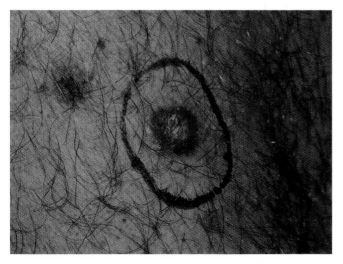

Fig. 3.87
Diagnosis: Dermatofibroma
Clinical Description: Firm, pink papule with peripheral pigment

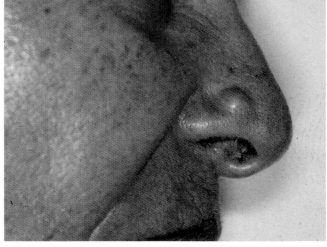

Fig. 3.90
Diagnosis: Lipoma
Clinical Description: Flesh-colored, mobile, subcutaneous nodule on the right nose

Fig. 3.91
Diagnosis: Keloid
Clinical Description: Pink, firm plaque

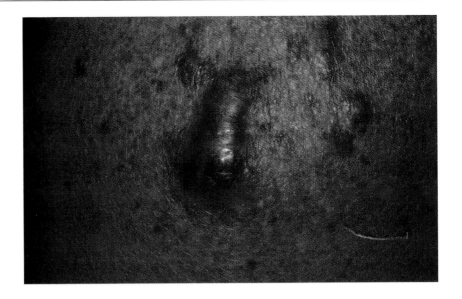

Fig. 3.92
Diagnosis: Cutaneous lupus
Clinical Description: Pink, scaly, plaque on left nasal dorsum

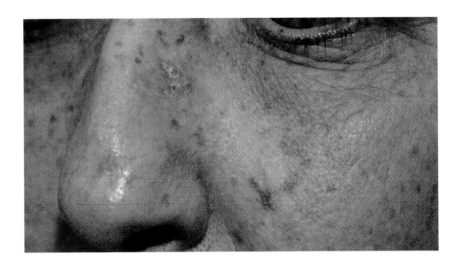

Fig. 3.93
Diagnosis: Cutaneous lupus
Clinical Description: Pink, eroded, scaly plaque on left conchal bowl

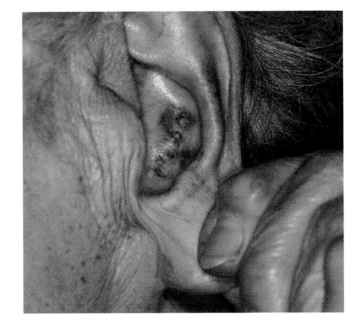

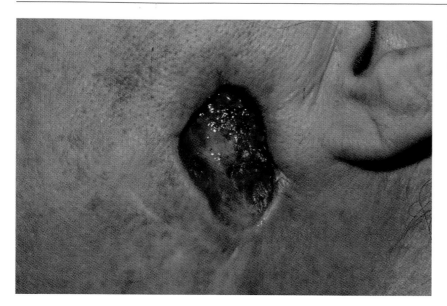

Fig. 3.94
Diagnosis: Factitial ulcer
Clinical Description: Sharply demarcated ulcer
with evidence of adjacent healed scars

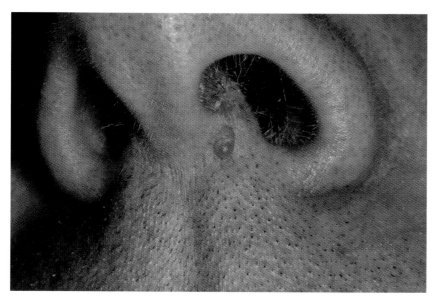

Fig. 3.95
Diagnosis: Angiofibroma
Clinical Description: Pink, opaque, dome-shaped
papule on left columella

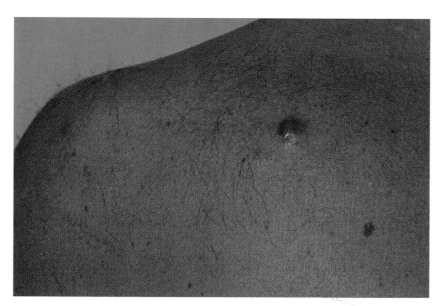

Fig. 3.96
Diagnosis: B cell lymphoma
Clinical Description: Pink plaque on left posterior
shoulder

Fig. 3.97
Diagnosis: Lymphomatoid papulosis
Clinical Description: Ulcerated, scaly plaque

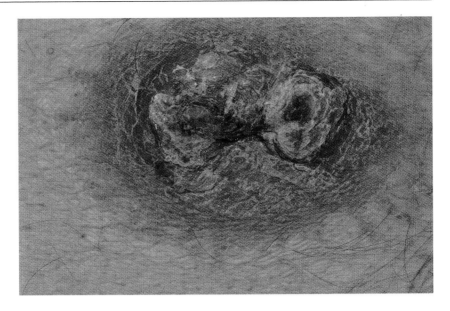

Fig. 3.98
Diagnosis: Nevus sebaceous
Clinical Description: Soft, pink-yellow papule on
the left cheek

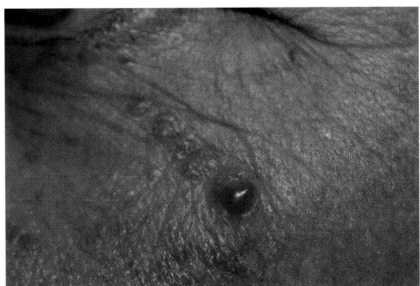

Fig. 3.99
Diagnosis: Xanthoma
Clinical Description: Pink plaque on forehead
with yellow margins on close inspection

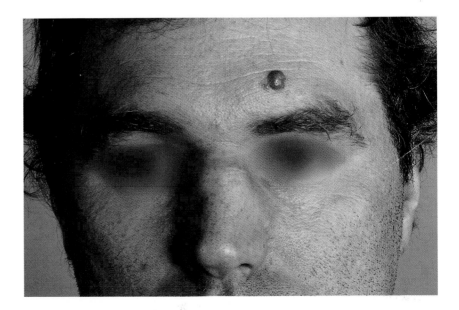

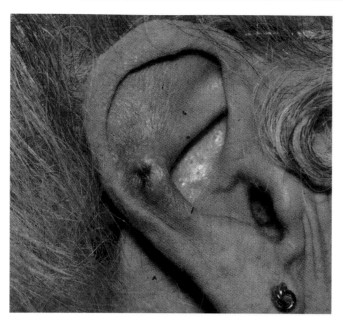

Fig. 3.100
Diagnosis: Chondrodermatitis nodularis chronica helicis (CNCH)
Clinical Description: Tender, pink, ulcerated papule overlying the cartilaginous antihelix

3.5 Clinical Images of SCC (Figs. 3.101–3.125)

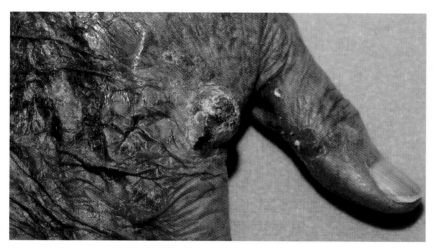

Fig. 3.101
Diagnosis: SCC -Keratoacanthoma type
Clinical Description: Keratotic nodule on the right hand

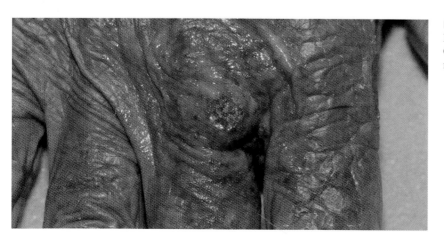

Fig. 3.102
Diagnosis: SCC-Keratoacanthoma type
Clinical Description: Keratotic, crateriform nodule on the right hand

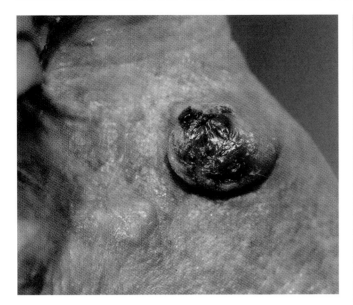

Fig. 3.103
Diagnosis: SCC-Keratoacanthoma type
Clinical Description: Keratotic papule on right nasal side wall

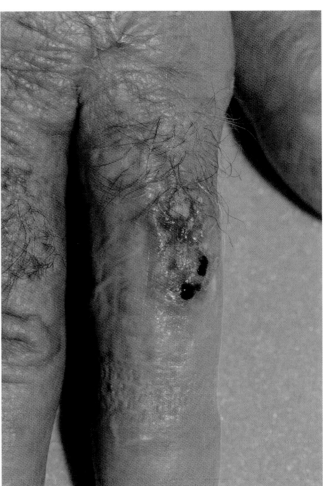

Fig. 3.105
Diagnosis: SCC
Clinical Description: Eroded ill-defined plaque on finger

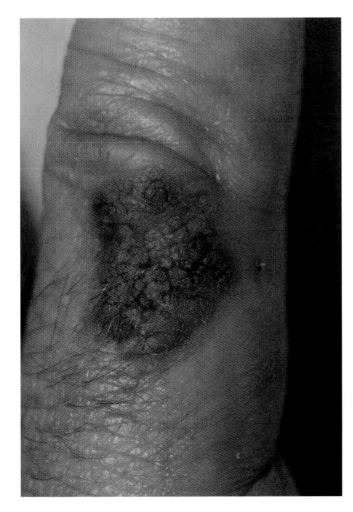

Fig. 3.104
Diagnosis: SCC in situ
Clinical Description: Scaly keratotic pink-brown plaque on finger

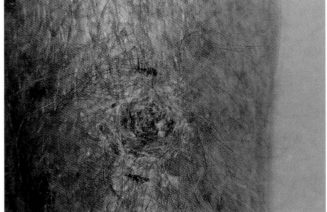

Fig. 3.106
Diagnosis: SCC
Clinical Description: Scaly keratotic plaque on skin

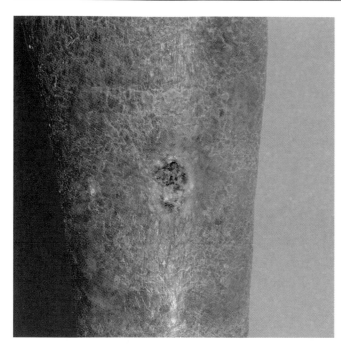

Fig. 3.107
Diagnosis: SCC
Clinical Description: Eroded scaly pink plaque on skin

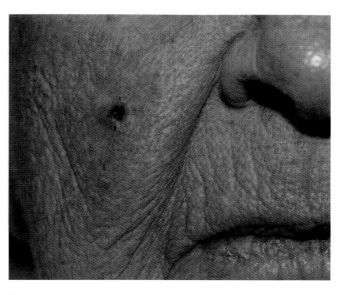

Fig. 3.109
Diagnosis: SCC
Clinical Description: pink eroded plaque on right cheek

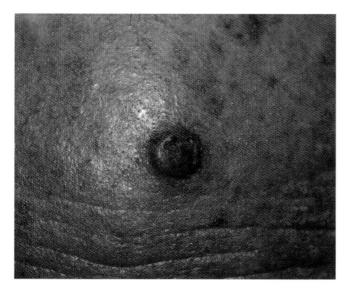

Fig. 3.108
Diagnosis: SCC
Clinical Description: Pink, keratotic papule on forehead

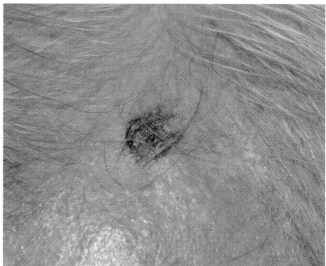

Fig. 3.110
Diagnosis: SCC
Clinical Description: Eroded scaly pink plaque on the scalp

Fig. 3.111
Diagnosis: SCC
Clinical Description: Dome-shaped ulcerated
plaque on the arm

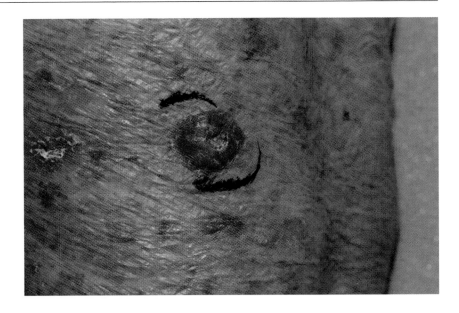

Fig. 3.112
Diagnosis: SCC in situ
Clinical Description: Pink scaly plaque on
left cheek

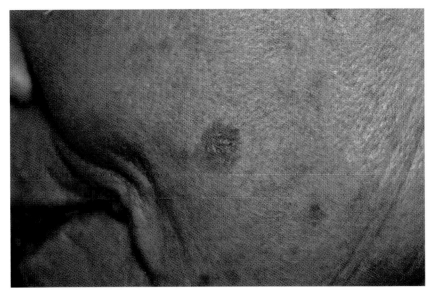

Fig. 3.113
Diagnosis: SCC
Clinical Description: Keratotic, crusted nodule
on the scalp

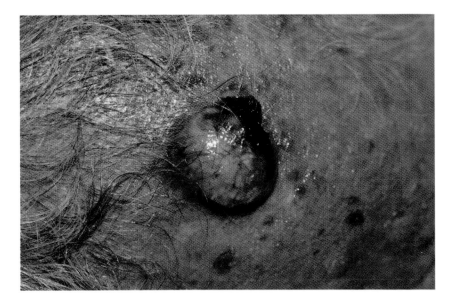

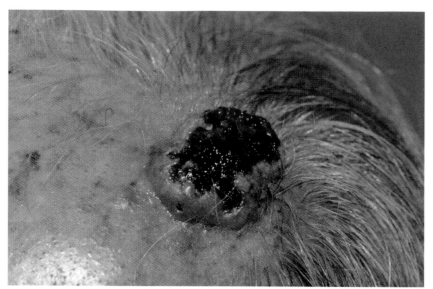

Fig. 3.114
Diagnosis: SCC
Clinical Description: Ulcerated, keratotic nodule
on the scalp

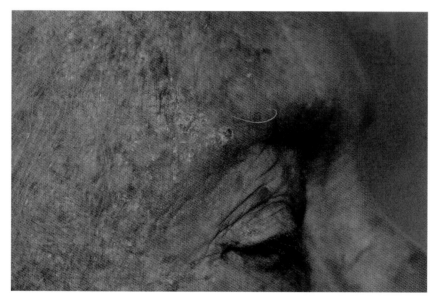

Fig. 3.115
Diagnosis: SCC
Clinical Description: Scaly pink plaque on right
lateral eyebrow

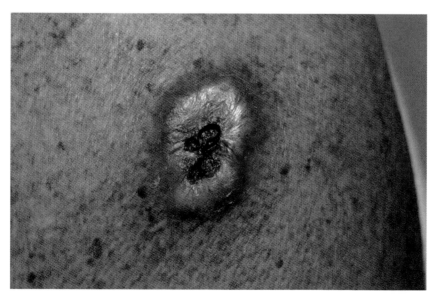

Fig. 3.116
Diagnosis: SCC
Clinical Description: Indurated, scaly plaque on
upper arm

Fig. 3.117
Diagnosis: SCC
Clinical Description: Scaly, keratotic plaque
below left ear

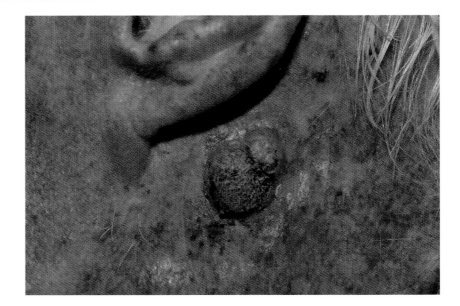

Fig. 3.118
Diagnosis: SCC
Clinical Description: Dome-shaped scaly plaque
on trunk

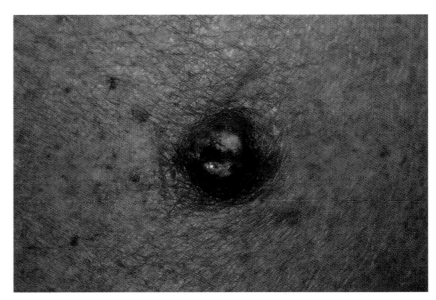

Fig. 3.119
Diagnosis: SCC
Clinical Description: Pink scaly plaque on the
lateral foot

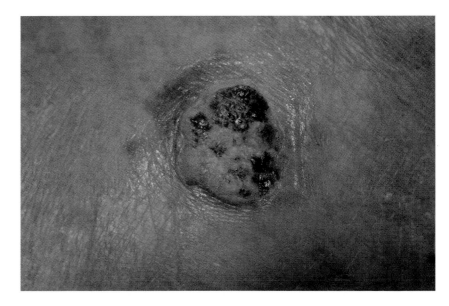

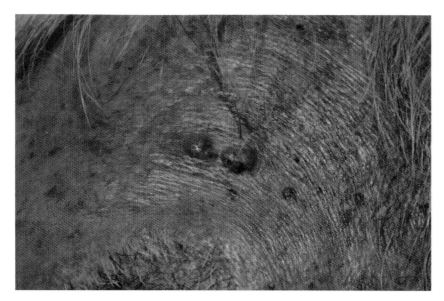

Fig. 3.120
Diagnosis: SCC x2
Clinical Description: Two firm papules on left forehead

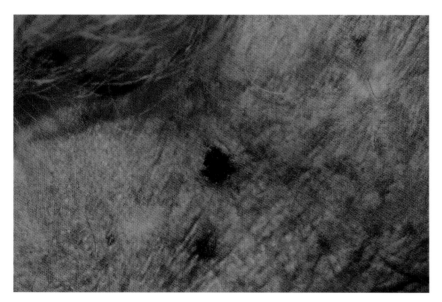

Fig. 3.121
Diagnosis: SCC
Clinical Description: Pink eroded plaque below right ear

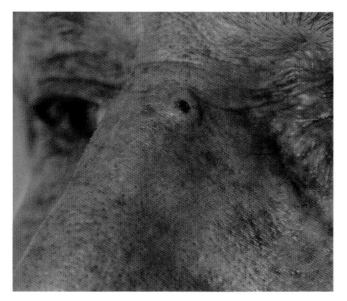

Fig. 3.122
Diagnosis: SCC
Clinical Description: Eroded papule on left upper nasal sidewall

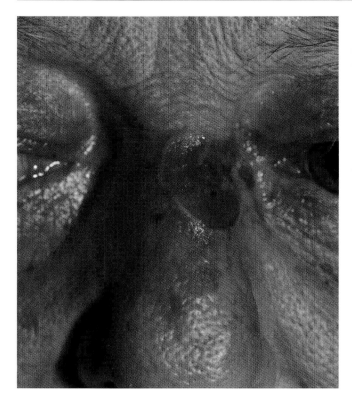

Fig. 3.123
Diagnosis: SCC
Clinical Description: Eroded pink plaque on nose

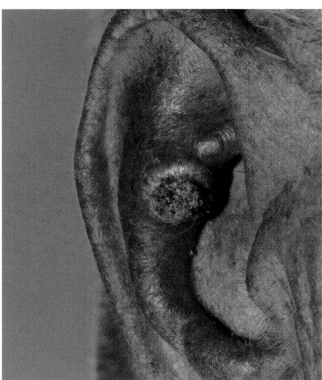

Fig. 3.125
Diagnosis: SCC-Keratoacanthoma type
Clinical Description: Keratotic, crateriform nodule with central debris on right antihelix of ear

3.6 Clinical Images of Mimickers of SCC (Figs. 3.126–3.139)

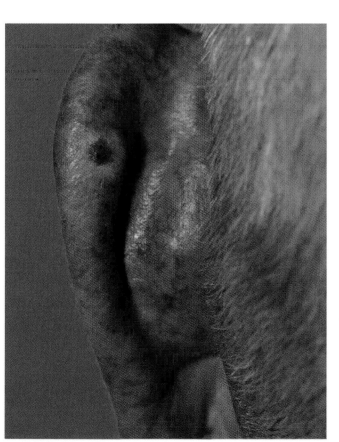

Fig. 3.124
Diagnosis: SCC
Clinical Description: Eroded pink plaque on left posterior helical rim

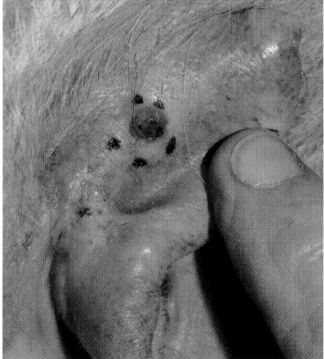

Fig. 3.126
Diagnosis: BCC
Clinical Description: Scaly pink plaque on right postauricular crease

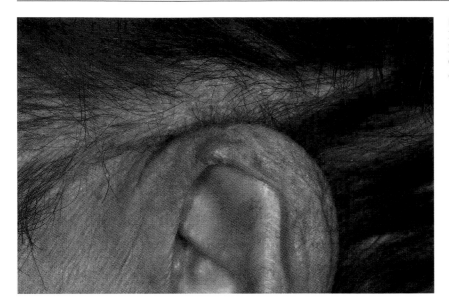

Fig. 3.127
Diagnosis: Chondrodermatitis nodularis
helicis (CNH)
Clinical Description: Tender pink papule
overlying helical cartilage

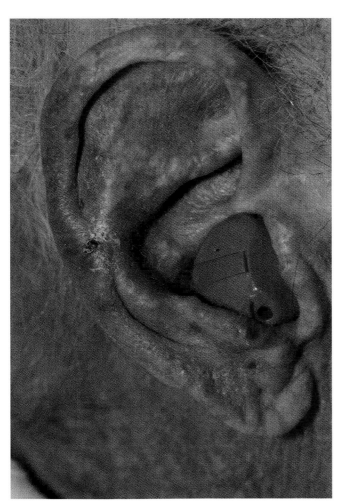

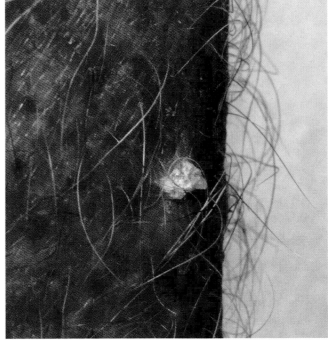

Fig. 3.128
Diagnosis: CNH
Clinical Description: Tender, eroded pink papule along helical rim

Fig. 3.129
Diagnosis: Cutaneous horn
Clinical Description: keratotic pink plaque on extremity

Fig. 3.130
Diagnosis: Factitial ulcers
Clinical Description: Multiple, superficial impetigenized ulcers on lower face

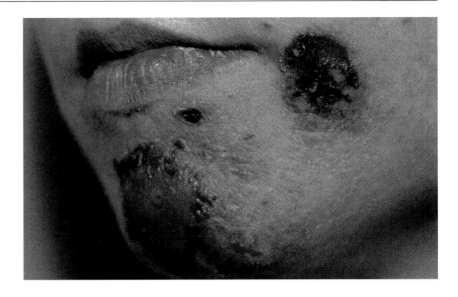

Fig. 3.131
Diagnosis: Lichen planus-hypertrophic
Clinical Description: Multiple scaly, pink papules

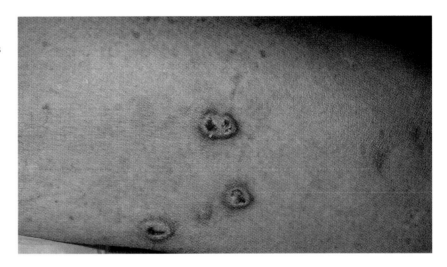

Fig. 3.132
Diagnosis: Insect bite
Clinical Description: Inflamed, scabbed, pink papule

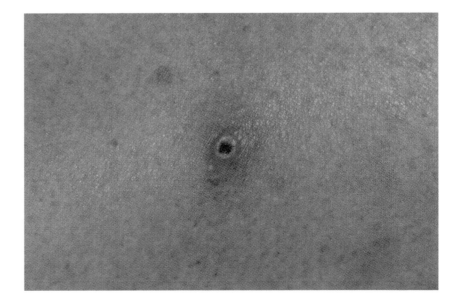

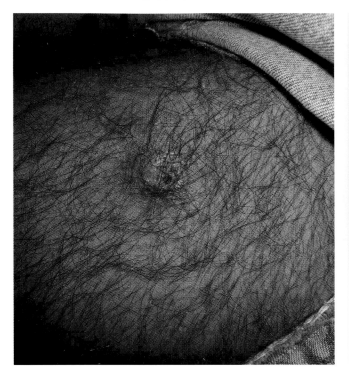

Fig. 3.133
Diagnosis: Kaposi sarcoma
Clinical Description: Violaceous, scaly plaque

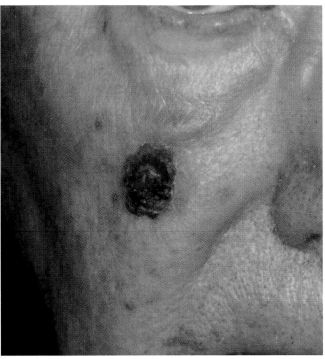

Fig. 3.135
Diagnosis: Merkel cell carcinoma
Clinical Description: Pink, scaly, crusted plaque on cheek

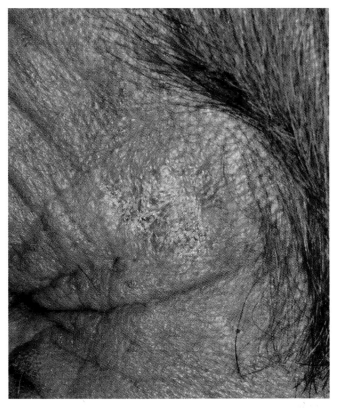

Fig. 3.134
Diagnosis: Cutaneous lupus
Clinical Description: Scaly crusted plaques on nose and lateral brow

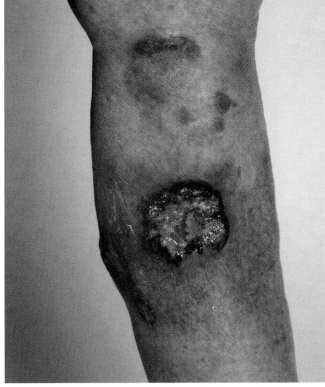

Fig. 3.136
Diagnosis: Mycosis fungoides
Clinical Description: Ulcerated pink plaques with violaceous borders

Fig. 3.137
Diagnosis: Molluscum contagiosum
Clinical Description: Small, pink, papule

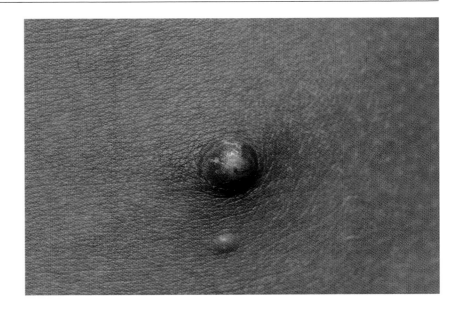

Fig. 3.138
Diagnosis: Porokeratosis
Clinical Description: Pink, scaly, plaque with peripheral
keratotic scale

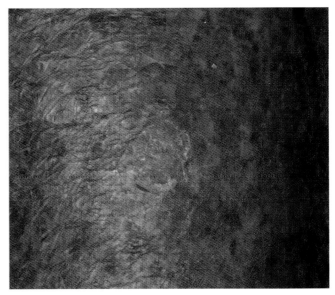

Fig. 3.139
Diagnosis: Prurigo nodularis
Clinical Description: Lichenified, pink, scaly
plaque

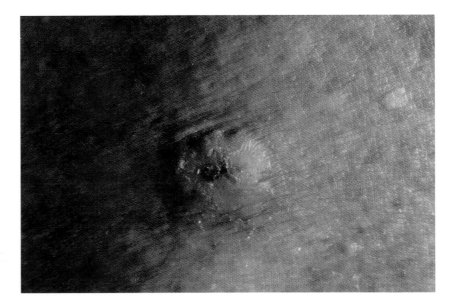

References

Brodland DG, Zitelli JA (1992) Surgical margins for excision of primary cutaneous squamous cell carcinoma. J Am Acad Dermatol 27(2 Pt 1):241–248

Christenson LJ, Borrowman TA, Vachon CM et al (2005) Incidence of basal cell and squamous cell carcinomas in a population younger than 40 years. JAMA 294:681–690

Gollnick H, Barona CG, Frank RG et al (2008) Recurrence rate of superficial basal cell carcinoma following treatment with imiquimod 5% cream: conclusion of a 5-year long-term follow-up study in Europe. Eur J Dermatol 18(6):677–682

Gross K, Kircik L, Kricorian G (2007) 5% 5-Fluorouracil cream for the treatment of small superficial basal cell carcinoma: efficacy, tolerability, cosmetic outcome, and patient satisfaction. Dermatol Surg 33(4):433–439

Marks R, Owens M, Walters SA et al (2004) Efficacy and safety of 5% imiquimod cream in treating patients with multiple superficial basal cell carcinomas. Arch Dermatol 140(10):1284–1285

Peris K, Campione E, Micantonio T et al (2005) Imiquimod treatment of superficial and nodular basal cell carcinoma: 12-week open-label trial. Dermatol Surg 31(3):318–323

Rodriguez-Vigil T, Vázquez-López F, Perez-Oliva N (2007) Recurrence rates of primary basal cell carcinoma in facial risk areas treated with curettage and electrodesiccation. J Am Acad Dermatol 56(1):91–95

Rowe DE, Carroll RJ, Day CL Jr (1989) Long-term recurrence rates in previously untreated (primary) basal cell carcinoma: implications for patient follow-up. J Dermatol Surg Oncol 15(3):315–328

Rowe DE, Carroll RJ, Day CL Jr (1992) Prognostic factors for local recurrence, metastasis, and survival rates in squamous cell carcinoma of the skin, ear, and lip. Implications for treatment modality selection. J Am Acad Dermatol 26(6):976–990

Tierney E, Barker A, Ahdout J et al (2009) Photodynamic therapy for the treatment of cutaneous neoplasia, inflammatory disorders, and photoaging. Dermatol Surg 35(5):725–746

Voss N, Kim-Sing C (1998) Radiotherapy in the treatment of dermatologic malignancies. Dermatol Clin 16(2):313–320

Wolf DJ, Zitelli JA (1987) Surgical margins for basal cell carcinoma. Arch Dermatol 123(3):340–344

4.1 Introduction

Malignant melanoma is the third most common type of skin cancer. Nevertheless, it is the leading cause of death due to skin cancer. Although melanoma can arise in many organs, the most common form, cutaneous melanoma, arises from the melanocytes that are found in the basal layer of the epidermis, hair follicles, sebaceous glands, and other adnexal structures.

Melanoma often presents as an irregularly bordered, pigmented macule. A melanoma presents with numerous shades of colors, ranging from tan to brown to jet-black, but they can also be evenly colored. Melanoma in situ, a variant of the disease which is confined to the epidermis, presents as a macule. Thin melanomas, those less than 1 mm in depth, often present in the same manner. Papular or nodular lesions are worrisome for deeper, more invasive disease. Finally, there is a non-pigmented variant referred to as amelanotic melanoma. This type of melanoma presents a diagnostic challenge and is often misdiagnosed at initial presentation.

The images in this chapter are meant emphasize to the reader both the hallmarks of melanoma and the great variability in its clinical presentation. All skin lesions suspicious for melanoma should be biopsied or referred for evaluation by a dermatologist. As mentioned above, melanoma is the leading cause of skin cancer-related death; early diagnosis and treatment saves lives.

4.2 Treatment of Melanoma

The standard treatment of melanoma remains surgical excision. A critical determinant of prognosis in melanoma is the Breslow thickness of the lesion, reported by the pathologist in millimeters. Recommended margins of excision are dependent on the thickness of the melanoma. Discussion of the full staging workup for a patient with melanoma is beyond the scope of this atlas but can be found in the National Comprehensive Cancer Networks (NCCN) Clinical Practice Guidelines in Oncology (2010).

Melanoma in situ carries a very low risk of metastasis. Standard of care for melanoma in situ on the trunk and extremities is local excision with 0.5 cm margins. Recent data suggest that melanoma in situ located on the head and neck, or in other chronically sun-exposed areas, requires margins greater than the suggested 0.5 cm for complete excision (National Comprehensive Cancer Network Clinical Practice Guidelines in Oncology 2010; Clark et al. 2008). Margin-controlled excision, which examines 100% of the surgical margin, offers the highest cure rates for melanoma in situ of the head and neck. This can be done using the Mohs technique with frozen sections and the with the aid of immunohistochemical stains, or with meticulously oriented permanent sections, a so-called staged excision. The cure rates associated with these techniques for the treatment of melanoma in situ ranges from 95% to 99% (Clark et al. 2008).

Invasive melanoma can carry significant risk of metastasis and death. The key prognostic factor for predicting the metastatic potential of a given primary tumor is its Breslow thickness. Likewise, the key prognostic factor for predicting overall survival in a given patient is sentinel lymph node status. Surgical excision of the primary tumor is the standard treatment for invasive melanoma. Sentinel lymph node biopsy should be considered in cases of invasive melanoma with a Breslow thickness greater than 1.0 mm. Referral to a physician who specializes in the management of melanoma is suggested for any patient with invasive melanoma.

A. Hendi and J.C. Martinez, *Atlas of Skin Cancers*,
DOI: 10.1007/978-3-642-13399-2_4, © Mayo Foundation for Medical Education and Research 2011

4.3 Clinical Images of Melanoma
(Figs 4.1–4.12)

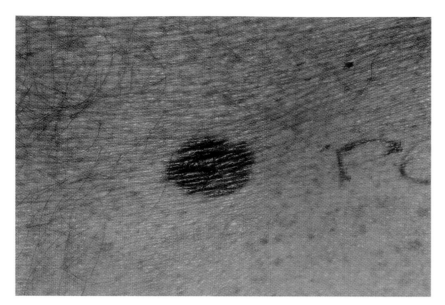

Fig. 4.1
Diagnosis: Superficial spreading melanoma
(1.0 mm Breslow thickness)
Clinical Description: Tan-brown pigmented
macule with irregular pigment and pink
discoloration

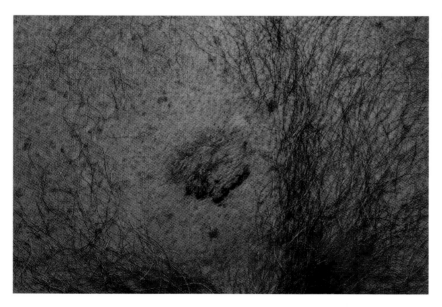

Fig. 4.2
Diagnosis: Superficial spreading melanoma
(0.9 mm Breslow thickness)
Clinical Description: Pink and gray
minimally elevated plaque with irregular
and hyperpigmented borders

Fig. 4.3
Diagnosis: Melanoma in situ
Clinical Description: Pink-brown tan macule
with irregular borders and color variegation

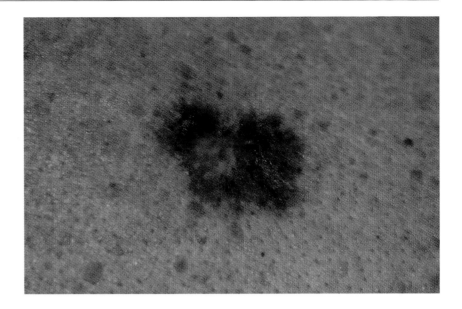

Fig. 4.4
Diagnosis: Nodular melanoma
Clinical Description: Reddish brown and
black nodule

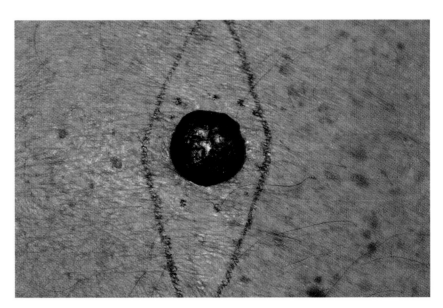

Fig. 4.5
Diagnosis: Melanoma in situ
Clinical Description: Pigmented macule with
irregular borders and color

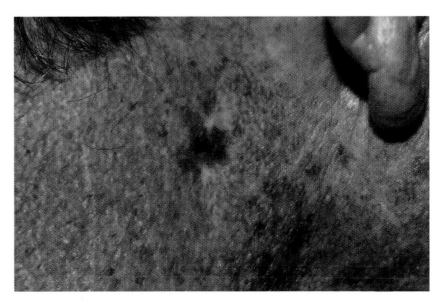

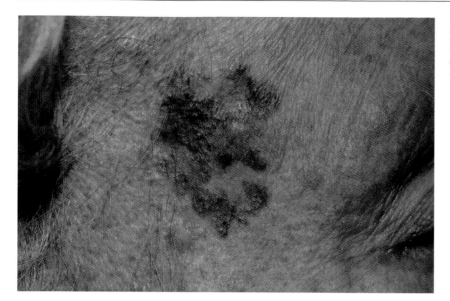

Fig. 4.6
Diagnosis: Superficial spreading melanoma
(<1 mm Breslow thickness)
Clinical Description: Large pigmented macule
with irregular borders

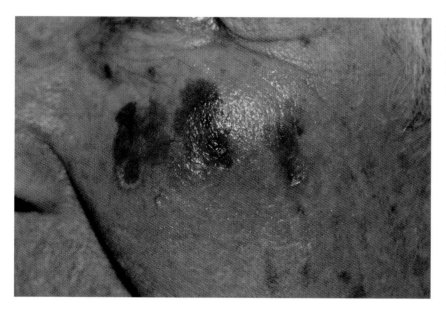

Fig. 4.7
Diagnosis: Melanoma in situ
Clinical Description: Large pigmented patch with
irregular borders and foci of hyperpigmentation.
Two areas of healing ulceration represent
biopsy sites

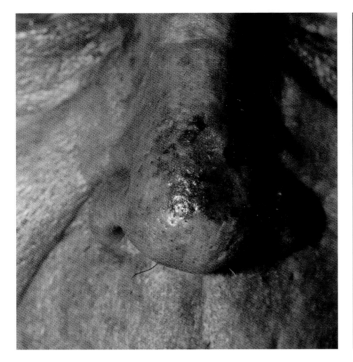

Fig. 4.8
Diagnosis: Melanoma in situ
Clinical Description: Pink-brown macule on nasal tip

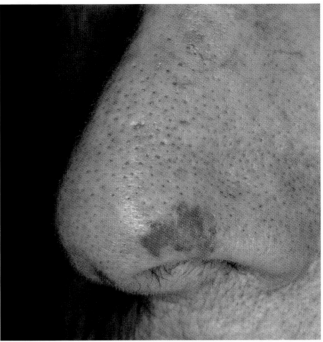

Fig. 4.10
Diagnosis: Amelanotic melanoma
Clinical Description: Pink minimally elevated plaque
left nasal alar rim

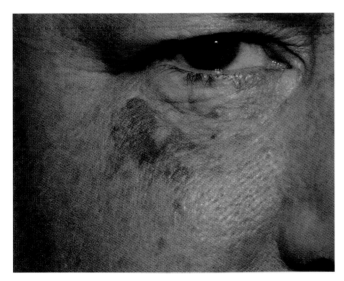

Fig. 4.9
Diagnosis: Melanoma in situ
Clinical Description: Pigmented macule on right infraorbital cheek

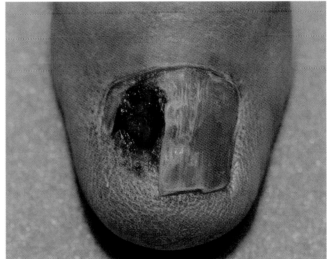

Fig. 4.11
Diagnosis: Amelanotic melanoma
Clinical Description: Erythematous, fleshy, subungual plaque

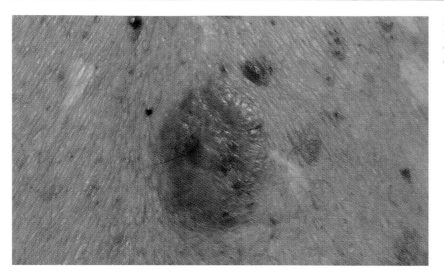

Fig. 4.12
Diagnosis: Amelanotic melanoma
Clinical Description: Pink plaque with minimal central pigmentation

4.4 Clinical Images of Mimickers of Melanoma (Figs 4.13–4.32)

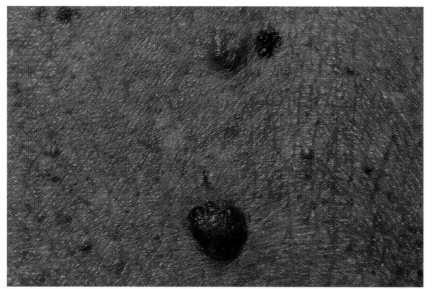

Fig. 4.13
Diagnosis: Benign Nevi
Clinical Description: Multiple nevi; Junctional nevus (*upper right*) – brown macule; dermal nevus (*upper left*) –tan papule; compound nevus (*mid lower*) – brown plaque

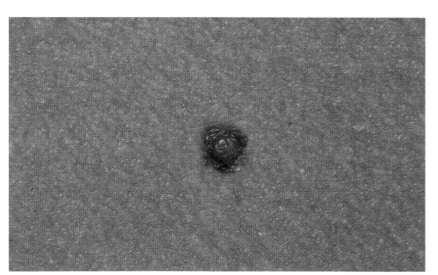

Fig. 4.14
Diagnosis: Benign compound nevus
Clinical Description: light brown papule with peripheral hyperpigmentation

Fig. 4.15
Diagnosis: Blue nevus
Clinical Description: Grayish blue papule

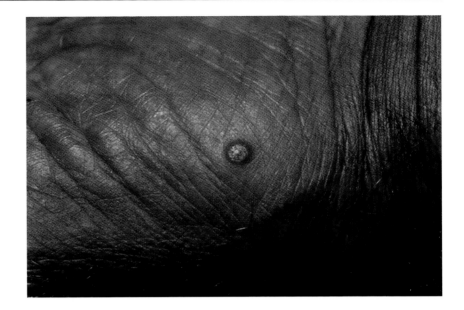

Fig. 4.16
Diagnosis: Blue nevus
Clinical Description: Blue macule on lower
lid margin

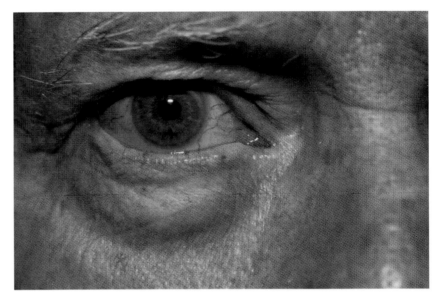

Fig. 4.17
Diagnosis: Congenital nevus
Clinical Description: Pigmented brown plaque
with focal areas of speckled hyperpigmentation

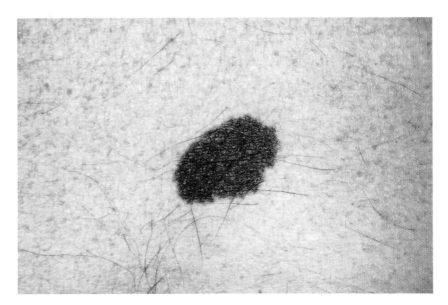

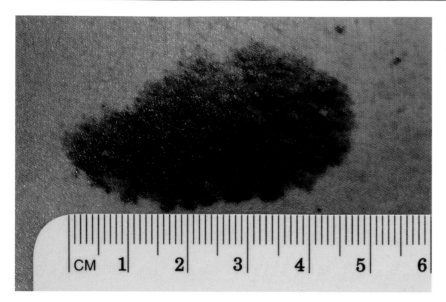

Fig. 4.18
Diagnosis: Congenital nevus
Clinical Description: Two toned oval-shaped plaque with irregular borders and speckled hyperpigmentation

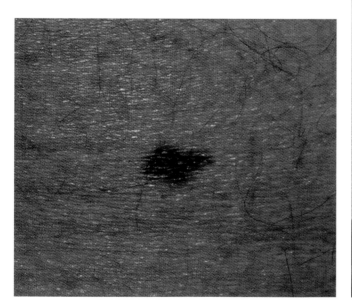

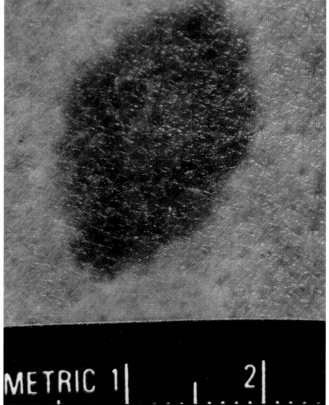

Fig. 4.19
Diagnosis: Dysplastic nevus
Clinical Description: reddish brown macule with irregular borders

Fig. 4.20
Diagnosis: Dysplastic nevus
Clinical Description: Two toned nevus with irregular borders

Fig. 4.21
Diagnosis: Seborrheic keratoses
Clinical Description: Multiple brown-black, stuck on-appearing papules and plaques

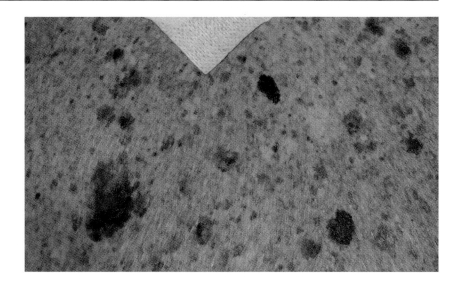

Fig. 4.22
Diagnosis: Seborrheic keratosis
Clinical Description: Tan-brown minimally elevated plaque on cheek

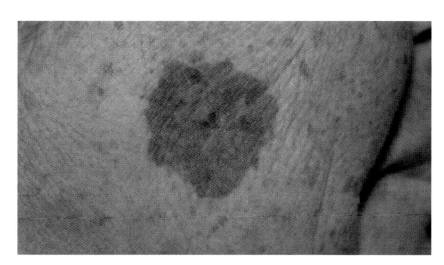

Fig. 4.23
Diagnosis: Melasma
Clinical Description: Pigmented irregular macule on cheek

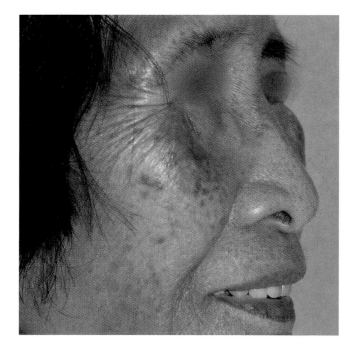

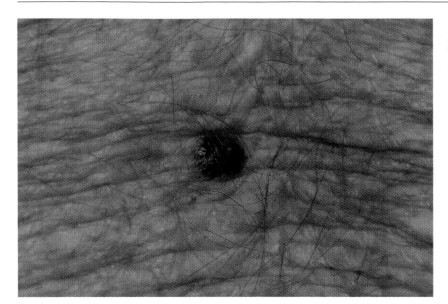

Fig. 4.24
Diagnosis: Pigmented BCC
Clinical Description: Brown papule with focal
areas of hyperpigmentation

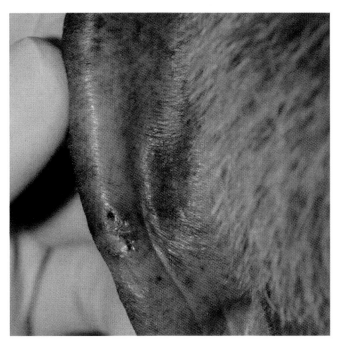

Fig. 4.25
Diagnosis: Pigmented BCC
Clinical Description: Pink-brown plaque on posterior helical rim

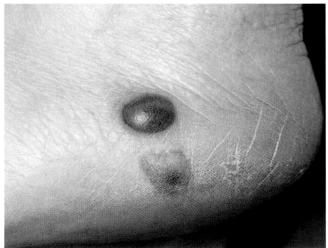

Fig. 4.26
Diagnosis: Hemorrhagic blister
Clinical Description: Two brown-black bullae on lateral aspect
of the left heel

Fig. 4.27
Diagnosis: Pyogenic granuloma
Clinical Description: Pink-black papule with
irregular coloration

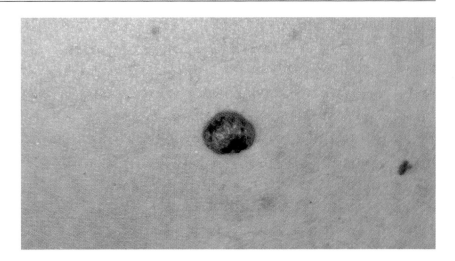

Fig. 4.28
Diagnosis: Follicular cyst – inflamed
(lower cheek lesion)
Clinical Description: Pink tender nodule on cheek

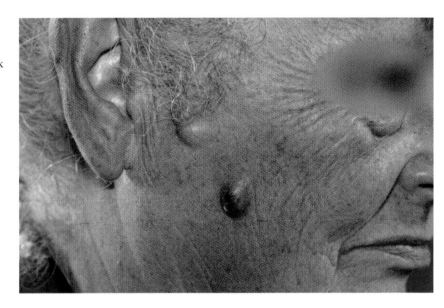

Fig. 4.29
Diagnosis: Pigmented actinic keratosis
Clinical Description: Minimally scaly,
hyperpigmented plaque with foci of uneven
coloration

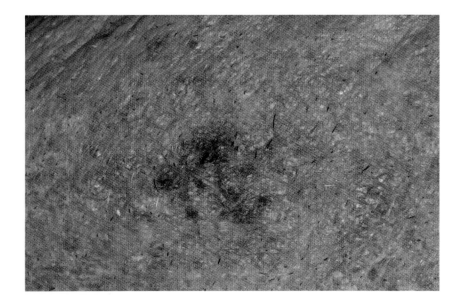

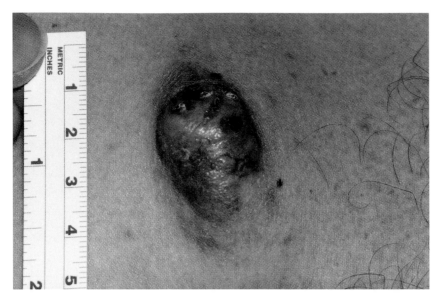

Fig. 4.30
Diagnosis: Dermatofibrosarcoma protuberans (DFSP)
Clinical Description: Firm, purplish, protuberant nodule

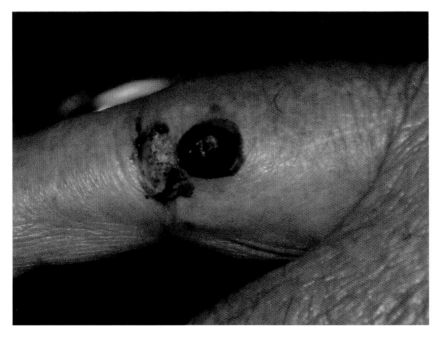

Fig. 4.31
Diagnosis: Thrombosed angiokeratoma
Clinical Description: black, hard papule adjacent to a friable, flesh-colored plaque

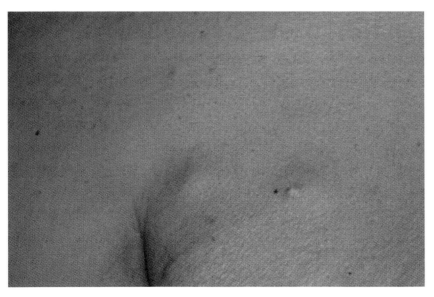

Fig. 4.32
Diagnosis: Glomus tumor
Clinical Description: deep, tender, hyperpigmented nodules on right buttock

References

Clark GS, Pappas-Politis EC, Cherpelis BS et al (2008) Surgical management of melanoma in situ on chronically sun-damaged skin. Cancer Control 15(3):216–224, 142(7):871–876

National Comprehensive Cancer Network Clinical Practice Guidelines in Oncology (2010) http://www.nccn.org/professionals/physician_gls/PDF/melanoma.pdf. Accessed 1.27.2010

Miscellaneous Cutaneous Neoplasms

5

Because of their low incidence and aggressive malignant potential, rare tumors such as atypical fibroxanthoma (AFX), dermatofibrosarcoma protuberans (DFSP), Merkel cell carcinoma, and sebaceous carcinoma are not discussed in greater detail in this atlas. For the sake of familiarization with the appearance of some of these benign and malignant neoplasms, the following images are included (Figs. 5.1–5.17).

Patients with these tumors should be referred to a physician who specializes in the management of uncommon cutaneous tumors for treatment and, if necessary, for further staging.

Fig. 5.1
Diagnosis: Hydrocystoma
Clinical Description: Flesh-colored cystic papules on right medial lower eyelid and medial canthus

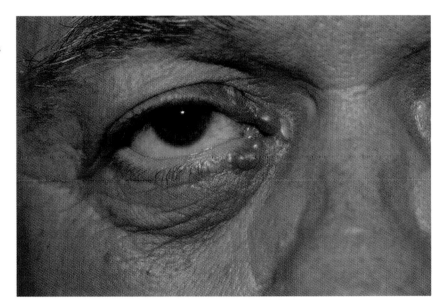

Fig. 5.2
Diagnosis: Trichilemmoma
Clinical Description: pink papule with central erosion on the left upper cutaneous lip

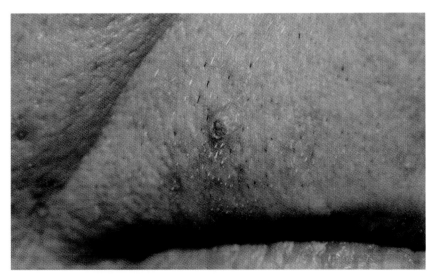

A. Hendi and J.C. Martinez, *Atlas of Skin Cancers*,
DOI: 10.1007/978-3-642-13399-2_5, © Mayo Foundation for Medical Education and Research 2011

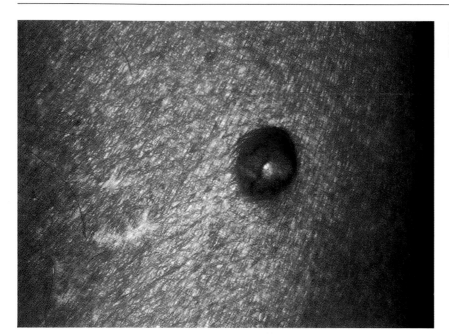

Fig. 5.3
Diagnosis: Spiradenoma
Clinical Description: Pink-purple, firm papule

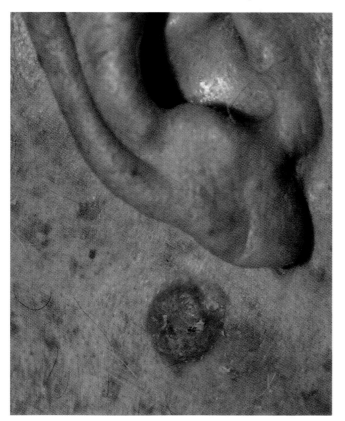

Fig. 5.4
Diagnosis: Atypical fibroxanthoma (AFX)
Clinical Description: Pink, scaly nodule on right infra-auricular neck

Fig. 5.5
Diagnosis: Porocarcinoma
Clinical Description: ulcerated, glistening nodular plaque replacing
right auricle (Photo courtesy of Jonathan L Cook, MD)

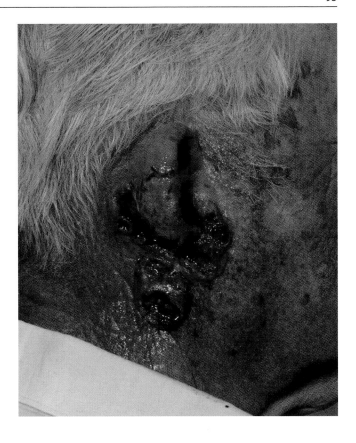

Fig. 5.6
Diagnosis: Dermatofibrosarcoma protuberans
(DFSP)
Clinical Description: Firm, ill-defined, scar-like
plaque

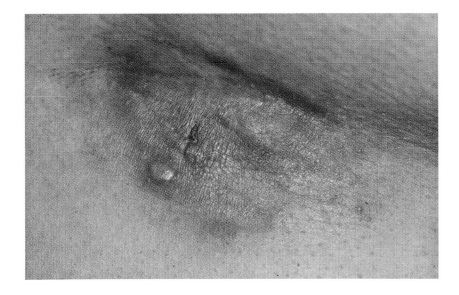

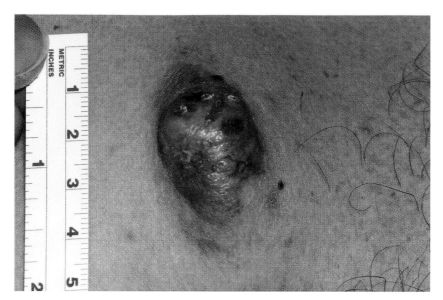

Fig. 5.7
Diagnosis: Dermatofibrosarcoma protuberans (DFSP)
Clinical Description: Violaceous, protuberant nodule

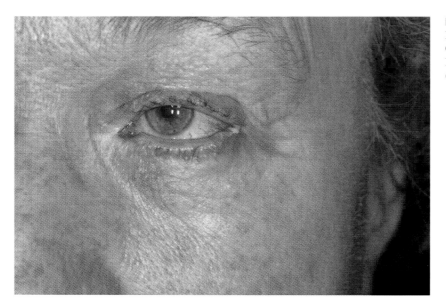

Fig. 5.8
Diagnosis: Sebaceous carcinoma
Clinical Description: Pink, eroded plaque on left lower lateral eyelid with loss of eyelashes (madarosis)

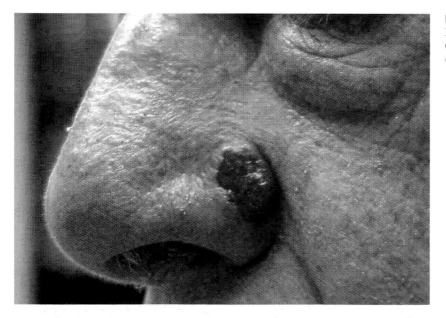

Fig. 5.9
Diagnosis: Sebaceous carcinoma
Clinical Description: Pink plaque on left nasal ala
(Photo courtesy of Jonathan L Cook, MD)

Fig. 5.10
Diagnosis: Extramammary Paget's disease
(EMPD)
Clinical Description: Ill-defined, pink, scaly patch
near the left inguinal fold

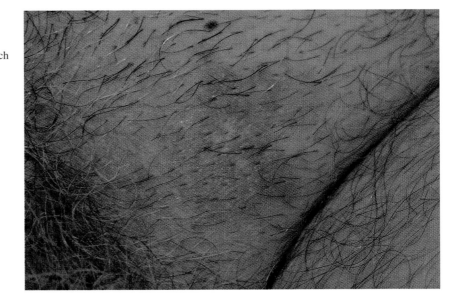

Fig. 5.11
Diagnosis: Extramammary Paget's disease
(EMPD)
Clinical Description: Ill-defined, pink, eroded
plaque on scrotum and base of penis

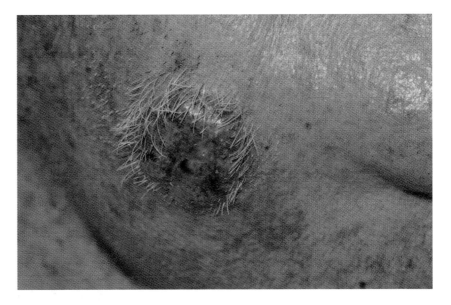

Fig. 5.12
Diagnosis: Merkel cell carcinoma
Clinical Description: Pink, pearly, telangiectatic
nodule without epidermal change

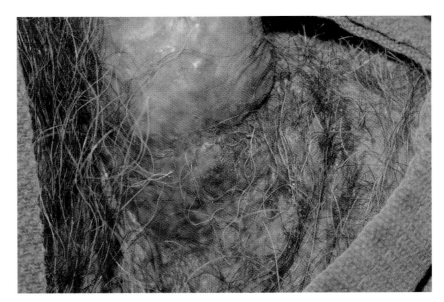

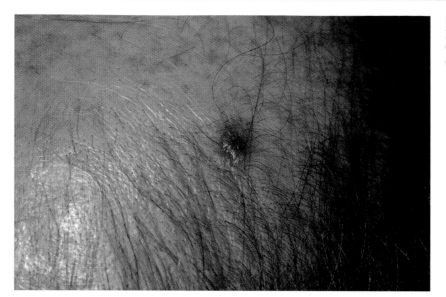

Fig. 5.13
Diagnosis: Pleomorphic undifferentiated sarcoma
Clinical Description: orange-red, smooth, nodule on scalp

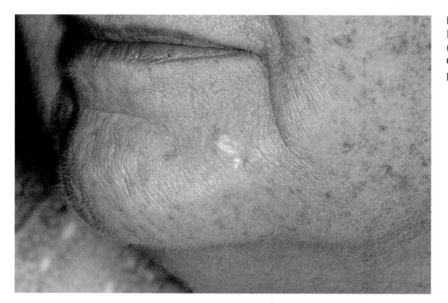

Fig. 5.14
Diagnosis: Microcystic adnexal carcinoma (MAC)
Clinical Description: Ill-defined, flesh-colored plaque on the left chin

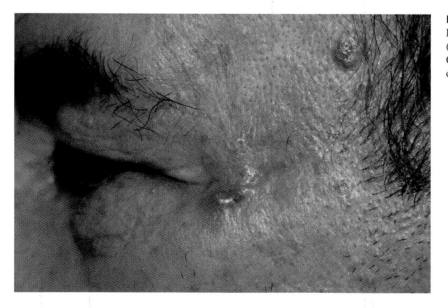

Fig. 5.15
Diagnosis: Microcystic adnexal carcinoma (MAC)
Clinical Description: Pink, ill-defined plaque on left temple

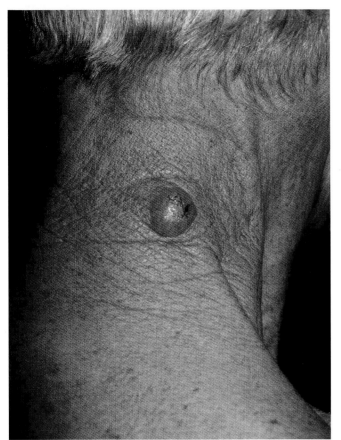

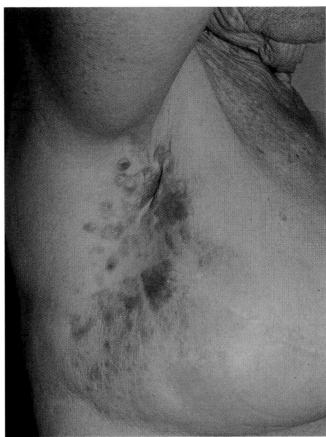

Fig. 5.16
Diagnosis: Squamous cell carcinoma – dermal metastasis
Clinical Description: Pink, hard, subcutaneous nodule on lateral neck

Fig. 5.17
Diagnosis: Metastatic breast cancer
Clinical Description: Coalescing pink, scaly plaques on right lateral
breast and axilla

6.1 Introduction

While clinical diagnosis may suffice for many lesions, biopsy is often required for confirmation of clinical suspicion and documentation purposes. This chapter will briefly describe several biopsy techniques and considerations. Wherever possible, photographic series clearly illustrating these techniques are included.

6.2 Local Anesthesia

It is important, for obvious reasons, to properly anesthetize the lesion of interest prior to biopsy. The anesthetic most commonly used is 1% lidocaine with 1:100,000 epinephrine. This can be buffered with bicarbonate to reduce the burning sensation during infiltration (Randle 1994). However, because the anesthetic is so fast-acting, the discomfort encountered with unbuffered anesthetic typically lasts only for 5–10 seconds.

Despite dogmatic teaching to the contrary, there is no good evidence that the addition of epinephrine to the numbing agent increases the risk of ischemic injury to distal sites such as the fingers, toes, the nose, or the penis. In fact, there is good evidence that this practice is perfectly safe (Krunic et al. 2004; Lalonde et al. 2005). The authors routinely use 1% lidocaine with 1:100,000 epinephrine to anesthetize all anatomic sites.

Patients complaining of an "allergy" or "reaction" to epinephrine seldom, if ever, have a true allergy to this naturally occurring substance. What many of these patients have most likely experienced in the past are palpitations, tachycardia, feelings of anxiety or panic, or temporary increase in blood pressure – the systemic effects of epinephrine. This systemic absorption from local anesthetic is much more commonly encountered with mucosal injections, such as those used at the dentist's office. If a patient complains only of this history, the authors commonly provide reassurance and proceed as per routine, as this reaction is essentially never encountered in patients receiving only 1.5–3 cc of intradermally or subcutaneously infiltrated 1% lidocaine with 1:100,000 epinephrine (Morganroth et al. 2009).

True allergy to lidocaine is rare and should be documented by an allergist on the patient's medical record. In the case of true allergy to lidocaine, there may be cross-reaction with any of the amide anesthetics, and local anesthesia may be obtained by injection of an esther anesthetic such as marcaine. Anesthesia may also be obtained, if not as predictably, with intradermal injection of preserved normal saline or with benzyl alcohol in preserved normal saline. Intradermal or subcutaneous injection with diphenhydramine has been suggested for anesthetic purposes in patients with lidocaine allergy. However, its manufacturers strongly discourage this practice, citing reports of local skin necrosis associated with cutaneous injection of intravenous diphenhydramine formulations.

A. Hendi and J.C. Martinez, *Atlas of Skin Cancers*,
DOI: 10.1007/978-3-642-13399-2_6, © Mayo Foundation for Medical Education and Research 2011

6.3 Numbing the Patient

Lesions should be marked at their clinical borders with a surgical marking pen, prior to numbing, as the tumescent and vasoconstrictive effects of local anesthetic can often make a subtle lesion vanish from the sight. If possible, only a single needlestick is used to anesthetize the entire area, and the needle is "fanned" under the lesion of interest while injecting the anesthetic. There is often immediate blanching of the skin around the defect due to both tumescent compression of small vessels and the vasoconstrictive properties of epinephrine.

Please see accompanying photographic series detailing infiltration of local anesthetic prior to biopsy (Figs. 6.1–6.5).

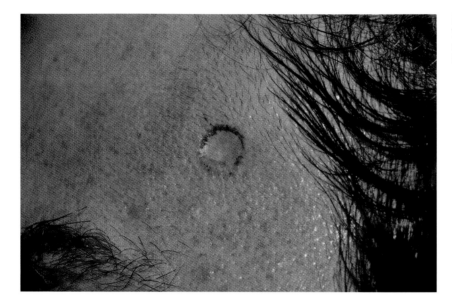

Fig. 6.1
The site is cleaned with alcohol, and the clinical margins of lesion to be biopsied are marked in indelible ink

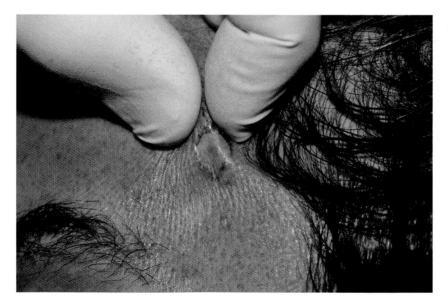

Fig. 6.2
The surrounding skin is pinched to "distract" from the sensation of needle entry

Fig. 6.3
The needle is inserted into the superficial dermis

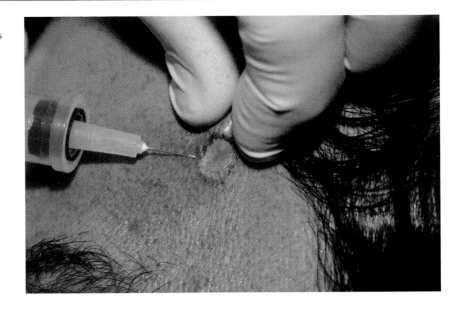

Fig. 6.4
An immediate blanching wheal is noted, verifying dermal, not subcutaneous, infiltration. Once this takes place, the needle may be advanced for subcutaneous infiltration as well

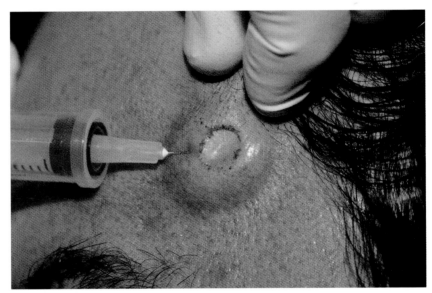

Fig. 6.5
Lesion is ready to be biopsied

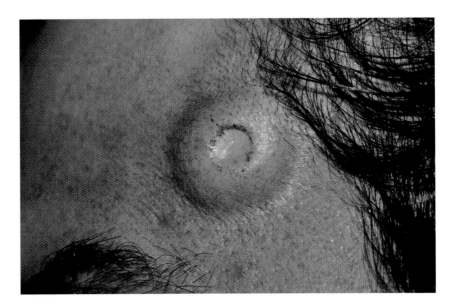

6.4 Shave Biopsy

This is perhaps the simplest and most common method of biopsy. This technique can be performed simply with either a scalpel or razor blade and is most commonly employed to biopsy a suspected epidermal or superficial dermal process. As such, is a great way to biopsy suspected nonmelanoma skin cancers (Figs. 6.6–6.14).

Care must be taken to include at least a small portion of the superficial dermis in order to detect invasive disease. The presence of pinpoint bleeding after biopsy will ensure that this level was reached. A biopsy report stating that the specimen was too superficial for diagnosis leads to awkward conversations with patients who now require a second biopsy to obtain a definitive diagnosis.

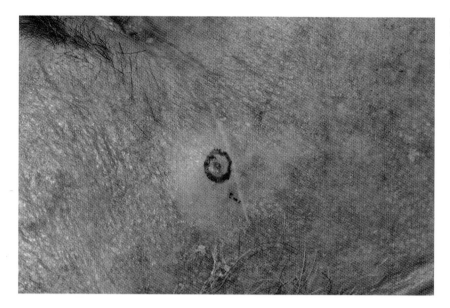

Fig. 6.6
The lesion to be biopsied is marked at its clinical borders with surgical marking pen and anesthetized as previously described

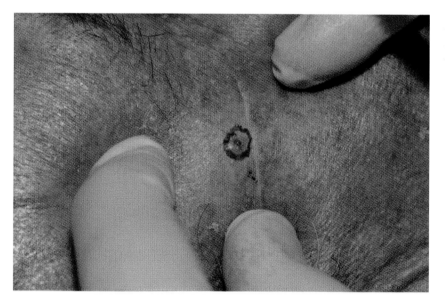

Fig. 6.7
Using two fingers of the nondominant hand, and fifth finger of the dominant hand, three point traction is placed, ensuring a taut surface

Fig. 6.8
The blade is held in the dominant hand and gently curved to allow for shallow shave biopsy

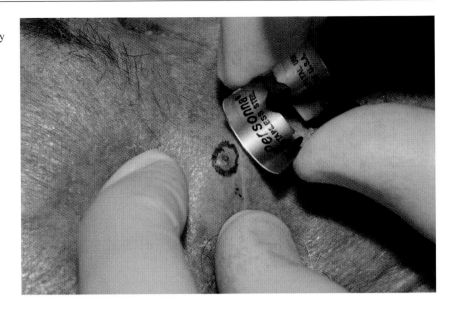

Fig. 6.9
Using a gentle side to side "sawing" motion, the edge of the blade is advanced under the lesion

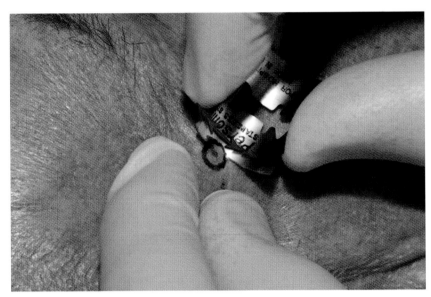

Fig. 6.10
The blade is brought back superficially at the distal edge of the lesion

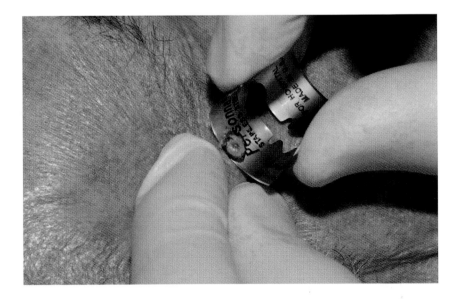

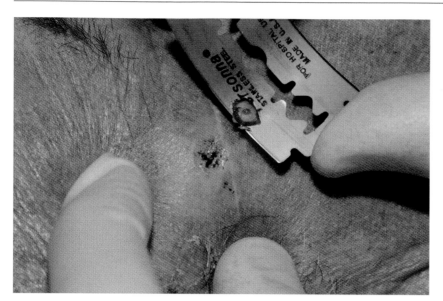

Fig. 6.11
Pinpoint bleeding demonstrates that the superficial dermis was reached on biopsy

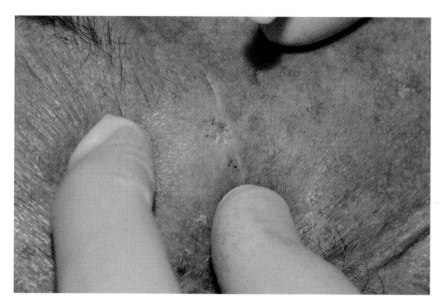

Fig. 6.12
The biopsy site is blotted dry and prepared for hemostasis and bandaging

Fig. 6.13
A cotton tip applicator dipped in 50% aluminum chloride is used to obtain hemostasis

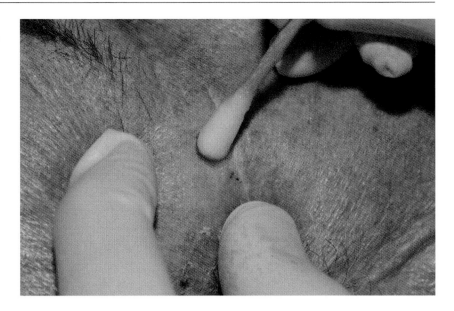

Fig. 6.14
The biopsy site is now ready to be bandaged

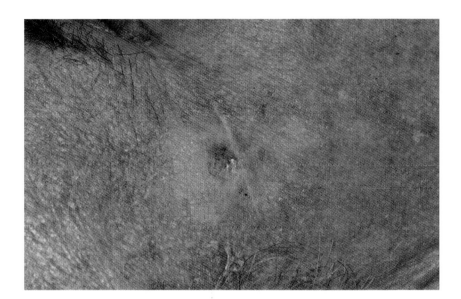

6.5 Punch Biopsy

Another common method used to biopsy cutaneous lesions is the punch biopsy. For this type of biopsy, a circular cookie cutter-like blade, called a trephine, is used. These are manufactured for single use and come in a variety of sizes, ranging from 2 to 10 mm. The most commonly used trephine is the 4-mm trephine, which allows for a small biopsy site scar, while almost always obtaining enough tissues for diagnosis. Measuring the lesion helps determine the correct size of trephine. Remember that, commonly, the purpose of the punch biopsy is merely to sample the lesion, and not necessarily to excise it in its entirety. The defect left by the biopsy is commonly sutured in a simple fashion; however, punch biopsies using a 4-mm trephine or a smaller one can be allowed to heal via second intention with no cosmetic penalty (Christenson et al. 2005) (Figs. 6.15–6.22).

When using the punch technique, it is important to consider and recognize what structures are underlying the biopsy site, as transection of an artery or cutaneous nerve is quite easy to do. In addition, care must be taken not to crush the tissue with the forceps, as this can impact the pathologist's ability to make a definitive diagnosis.

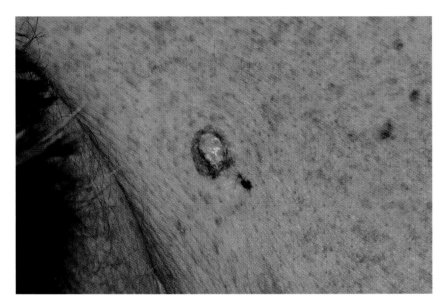

Fig. 6.15
The lesion to be biopsied is marked at its clinical borders with surgical marking pen and anesthetized as previously described

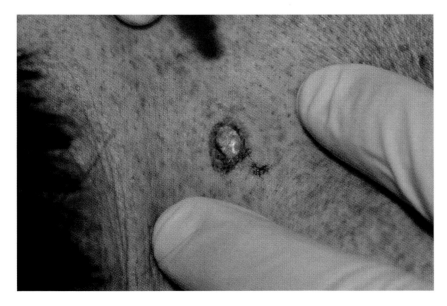

Fig. 6.16
Using two fingers of the nondominant hand, and the fifth finger of dominant hand, three point traction is placed, ensuring a taut surface

Fig. 6.17
While rolling the trephine between the thumb and forefinger of the dominant hand, downward pressure is applied, until the desired depth is reached

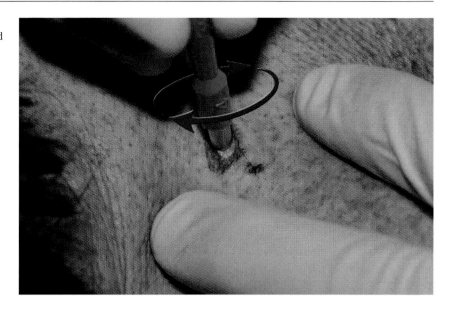

Fig. 6.18
The tissue sample appears to "float" in the defect once it has been detached from surrounding dermis

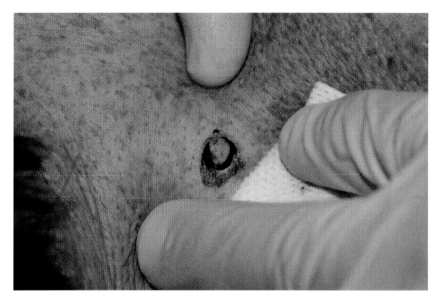

Fig. 6.19
While gently grasping and lifting the tissue with forceps, sharp scissors are used to snip the tissue free from the attached subcutaneous fat

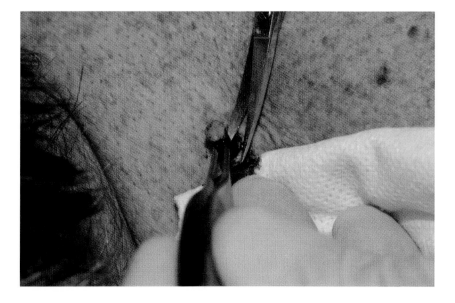

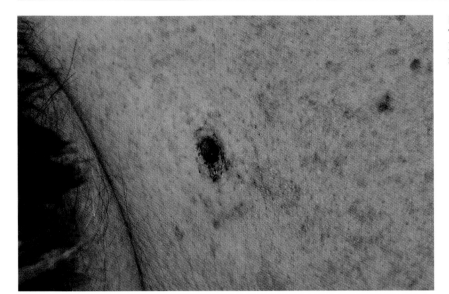

Fig. 6.20
The specimen has been removed and placed in a labeled formalin-filled container. The defect is ready to be sutured

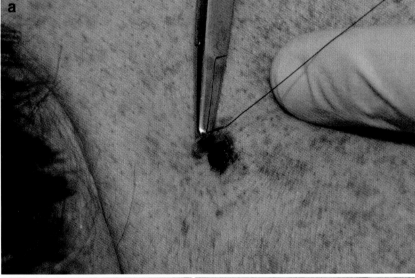

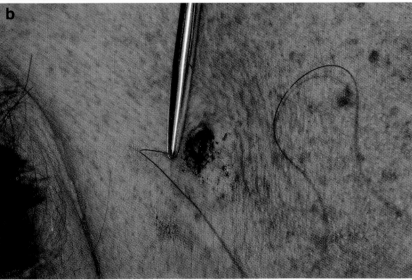

Fig. 6.21
(**a–d**) A figure-of-eight suture is placed using nylon suture

Fig. 6.21
(continued)

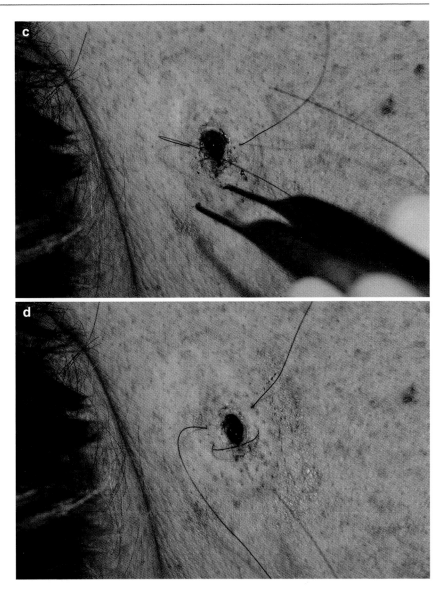

Fig. 6.22
The biopsy site is ready for bandaging

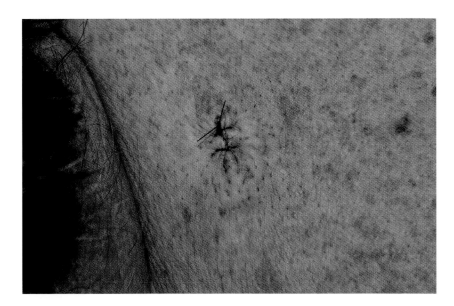

6.6 Excisional Biopsy

An excisional biopsy is simply the complete removal of an undiagnosed lesion. The edges of the lesion are identified clinically, and the appropriate margins are delineated with a surgical marking pen. The area to be excised is then anesthetized as detailed above and the biopsy is carried out as illustrated in the accompanying photographic series below.

If the lesion is quite small (2–5 mm), an appropriately sized trephine can be used to entirely excise the lesion (Figs. 6.23–6.31).

For lesions larger than 5–6 mm, an excisional biopsy is often performed. There is no difference between this biopsy and an excision except that the lesion has not yet been diagnosed (see Sect. 3.2.3).

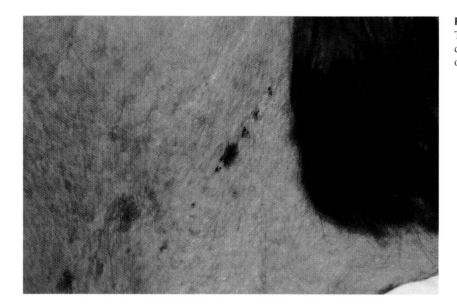

Fig. 6.23
The lesion is identified and anesthetized. Inked dots are used here to illustrate the planned orientation of closure

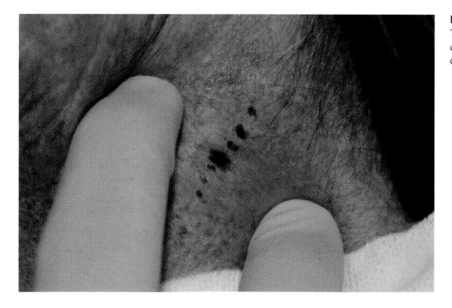

Fig. 6.24
Traction is applied perpendicular to the planned closure direction. Note stretching of the inked dots and of the pigmented lesion

Fig. 6.25
While still applying traction, the skin is scored
with the trephine

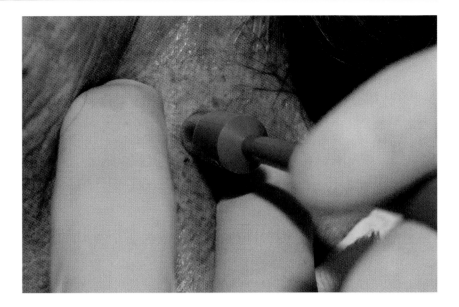

Fig. 6.26
The site is checked after scoring to ensure that the
lesion will be entirely removed by the proposed
excision of tissue. The trephine is then inserted
to the depth of the subcutaneous fat to ensure
adequate excision

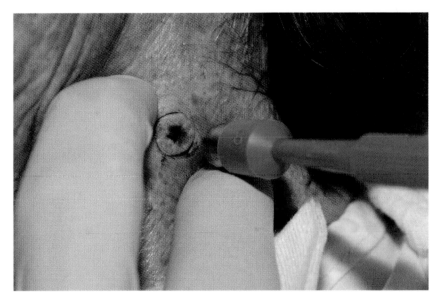

Fig. 6.27
Releasing traction allows tissue to regain
"normal" configuration. The specimen is gently
lifted with forceps to allow removal with scissors

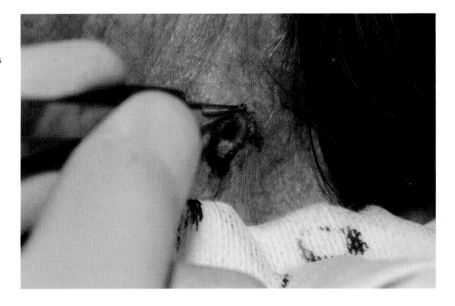

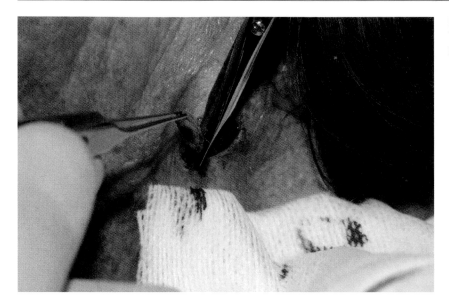

Fig. 6.28
The specimen is removed, ensuring that no
pigment is seen at base of tissue

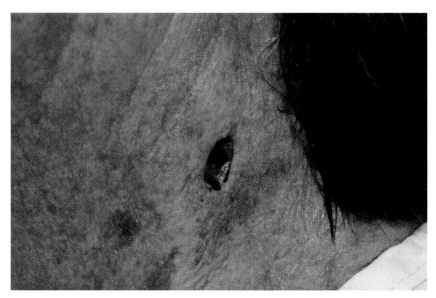

Fig. 6.29
Note that the circular defect has assumed an
elliptical shape along the planned axis of closure

Fig. 6.30
A single deep-buried suture is placed. Note the complete dermal and epidermal closure along planned axis

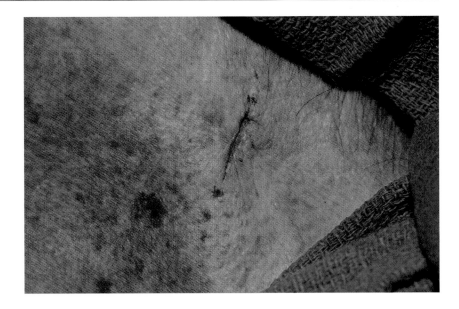

Fig. 6.31
Top stitches are then placed to seal epidermal edges

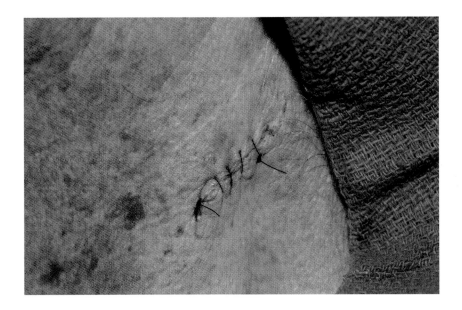

6.7 Incisional Biopsy

An incisional biopsy refers simply to the fact that the biopsy is not removing the lesion in its entirety. This can be done for lesions that are too large to be removed feasibly with a single biopsy procedure; for example, an 8 cm pigmented macule on a patient's scalp (Fig. 6.32). An area felt to be representative of the entire lesion is then selected and outlined using a surgical marking pen. That area is then excised and closed primarily as detailed and illustrated in Chap. 3.

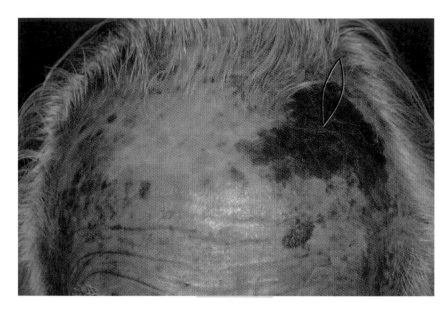

Fig. 6.32
Schematic detailing planned elliptical incisional biopsy

6.8 Anatomic Locations

Certain anatomic locations require more care when performing a biopsy. Especially for biopsies performed on the face, patients may often have cosmetic concerns. There is a balance between removing enough tissue to obtain a diagnostic biopsy and taking too much tissue. If no further treatment is required after biopsy, the biopsy site will usually heal as an atrophic, hypopigmented, depressed scar. Care should be taken, especially with facial biopsies, to minimize cosmetic impact of a biopsy in case no further treatment is required. Regardless of anatomic location, suspicious pigmented lesions should be biopsied excisionally if at all possible. A biopsy showing a melanoma transected at its base fails to provide an accurate assessment of thickness – a critical determinant of prognosis.

6.9 Wound Care

Wound care for biopsy sites is quite straightforward. Usually, petrolatum and either a small pressure bandage or a simple adhesive bandage are placed at the time of biopsy. This bandage can stay on for 24 hours. After that, the area is gently cleansed two to three times daily with soap and water. After each cleaning, a small amount of petrolatum and a fresh bandage are applied. Some surrounding redness, swelling, and tenderness are to be expected for the first 2 or 3 days. Persistent or increasing discomfort and swelling should raise suspicion of a biopsy site infection.

Any sutures placed at the time of biopsy should be removed at the physician's discretion. The authors usually remove sutures at 1 week from the face, trunk, and upper extremities and at 2 weeks on the lower extremities.

References

Christenson LJ, Phillips PK, Weaver AL, Otley CC (2005) Primary closure vs second-intention treatment of skin punch biopsy sites: a randomized trial. Arch Dermatol 141(9):1093–1099

Krunic AL, Wang LC, Soltani K et al (2004) Digital anesthesia with epinephrine: an old myth revisited. J Am Acad Dermatol 51(5):755–759

Lalonde D, Bell M, Benoit P et al (2005) A multicenter prospective study of 3, 110 consecutive cases of elective epinephrine use in the fingers and hand: the Dalhousie Project clinical phase. J Hand Surg Am 30(5):1061–1067

Morganroth PA, Gelfand JM, Jambusaria A et al (2009) A randomized, double-blind comparison of the total dose of 1.0% lidocaine with 1:100,000 epinephrine versus 0.5% lidocaine with 1:200,000 epinephrine required for effective local anesthesia during Mohs micrographic surgery for skin cancers. J Am Acad Dermatol 60(3):444–452

Randle HW (1994) Reducing the pain of local anesthesia. Cutis 53(4):167–170

7.1 Introduction

Treatment of skin cancers has an inherent risk of complications, as with any other medical treatment. The main complications seen with the surgical treatment of skin cancers are the same as with any other surgery. They include infection, bleeding, dehiscence, and necrosis. These four interrelated complications are often referred to as the "terrible tetrad" (Hendi 2007). The rate of these complications is relatively low with dermatologic surgery procedures (Cook and Perone 2003; Aasi and Leffell 2003).

7.2 Terrible Tetrad

Bleeding can be the most serious complication of the "terrible tetrad." Bleeding as a complication can be attributed to inadequate intraoperative hemostasis, coagulopathy, poor pressure dressing, and exertion by the patient, or manipulation of the surgical site. Wounds that are allowed to granulate, either after surgery or a simple ED&C procedure, will often ooze serous or serosanguinous fluid for several days after the procedure. Frank bleeding, if it is going to occur, will usually manifest early on. However, delayed bleeding can be seen in patients on anticoagulant medications. If the bleeding is minor, it can usually be successfully managed by application of continuous pressure by the patient for 30 min. If this is not effective, the bleeding should be evaluated by a healthcare provider. Pinpoint bleeding can be managed by cauterization of the blood vessels under local anesthesia, while arterial bleeding may require suture ligations.

Bleeding that occurs under a sutured wound can lead to hematoma formation. A hematoma can be acute or expanding, which requires surgical intervention, or stable and self-limited. An acute hematoma occurs within hours after surgery (Fig. 7.1). Patients will often complain of sudden onset of throbbing pain, and evaluation of the surgical site reveals significant bruising and swelling of the surgical site. The treatment of an acute or expanding hematoma is to open the wound, visualize the source of the bleeding, and obtain hemostasis either by suture

ligation of the bleeding vessel or electrocautery. Stable hematomas usually present several days after surgery (Fig. 7.2). These are self-limited hematomas, where the postoperative bleeding stops due to the tamponade effect of the hematoma on the bleeding vessel(s). Such hematomas undergo an evolution process, which leads to the resolution of the hematoma in several weeks. Most stable hematomas can be treated conservatively by observation or aspiration. Patients with either type of hematomas are generally treated with antibiotics as the devitalized, extravascular blood under skin can be a nidus for

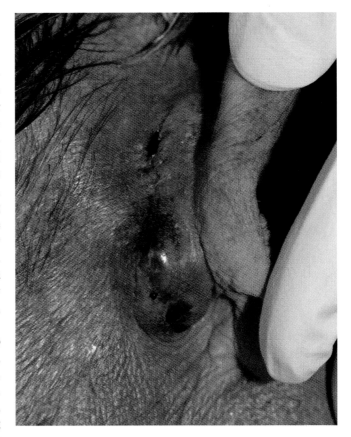

Fig. 7.1
Acute hematoma on the post auricular crease presenting within 24 hours after surgery

A. Hendi and J.C. Martinez, *Atlas of Skin Cancers*,
DOI: 10.1007/978-3-642-13399-2_7, © Mayo Foundation for Medical Education and Research 2011

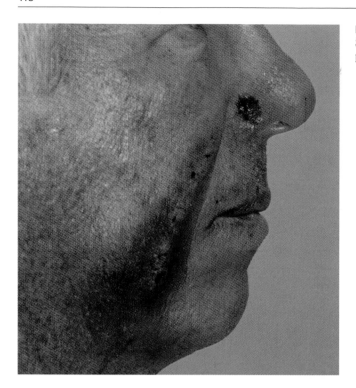

Fig. 7.2
Stable hematoma on the lower cheek presenting at the 1-week
post-op visit

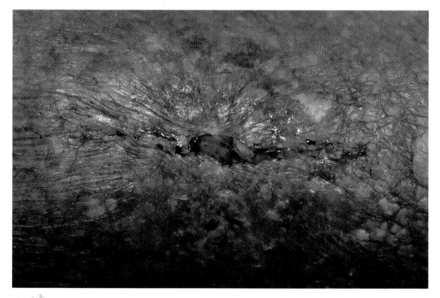

Fig. 7.3
Wound infection on arm. Note purulent discharge

an infection. Surgical techniques that minimize the incidence
of hematoma formation include meticulous pinpoint cautery,
and suture ligation of arterial bleeding points.

Infection after skin surgery is relatively uncommon and
should occur in less than 5% of cases. Postoperative infection
is often noted 5–7 days after surgery and is commonly associated with *increasing* redness, pain, swelling, and warmth.
Purulent drainage from the surgical wound (Fig. 7.3) and systemic symptoms such as fever and malaise may also be

present. The causes of postoperative infection can be divided
into technique-related or patient-related factors. Technique-
related factors include inadequate surgical prep/contamina-
tion, traumatic tissue handling (i.e., with forceps), excess
cautery, excess tension, and presence of dead space, which
can lead to hematoma formation. Patient-related factors
include inadequate postoperative wound care and coloniza-
tion by higher than normal number of normal skin flora
(*Staphylococcus aureus*) or other pathogenic bacteria (i.e.,

MRSA). Patients with psoriasis, eczema, seborrheic dermatitis, or dry/scaly skin are often colonized by a higher than normal number of skin flora. Petroleum ether or rubbing alcohol can be used to remove the scaly skin around the surgical site prior to surgery. Certain sites, such as the lower extremities, have a higher likelihood of postoperative infection. *All* wound infections should be cultured and treated with antibiotics, which can later be adjusted, based on the sensitivity results. It is important to allow for drainage of pus after a wound infection. With open wounds, this takes place naturally. Sutured wounds may need to be partially opened to allow for drainage of pus, unless the infection is diagnosed early and the wound is not fluctuant.

There are several conditions that may mimic a surgical site infection. The initial stages of wound healing, the inflammatory phase, is associated with erythema, minor swelling, and warmth, and should not be confused with an infection. Contact dermatitis at the surgical site may be associated with redness, swelling, and drainage similar to an infection (Fig. 7.4). However, contact dermatitis is not associated with increasing pain, and is often accompanied instead by itching.

Dehiscence is the separation of sutured wound edges (Fig. 7.5a, b). This is more commonly a manifestation of poor healing at the wound edges. Technique-related causes include excess tension/inadequate undermining, inadequate suture selection, and early suture removal. Patient-related causes include early postoperative exertion or trauma to the wound. Yet, the most common causes of dehiscence include infection, necrosis, and hematoma, the other members of the "terrible tetrad." Early and large wound dehiscence (i.e., post-op days 1–2) can be re-sutured under sterile conditions. Small/superficial or late wound dehiscence can be allowed to heal by second intention.

Necrosis can be seen at the edges of a closure (Fig. 7.6a, b). This can occur if the wound is closed under significant tension, or at the distal tip of a flap. As with the other complications, the causes of necrosis can be divided into technique-related and patient-related causes. The technique-related causes include excess tension on the wound margins (due to improper/inadequate undermining or suturing the wound edges too tightly) or poor flap design. In addition, hematoma and infection can also lead to necrosis. Patient-related causes include smoking, location (such as the legs), arterial disease, and history of radiation. Heavy smokers (more than one pack per day) are believed to have a higher risk of necrosis (Goldminz and Bennett 1991). Although a recent study refutes this, the amount of smoking was not accounted for in this study (Dixon et al. 2009). Postoperative wound necrosis can be managed conservatively with daily moist dressings.

7.3 Miscellaneous Complications

Less common surgical complications include suture granuloma and epidermal maturation arrest (Hendi 2008). Suture granuloma or abscess present as a pink, tender papule or cystic lesion within the incision line 4–6 weeks after

Fig. 7.4
Contact dermatitis to triple antibiotic ointment used on surgical site

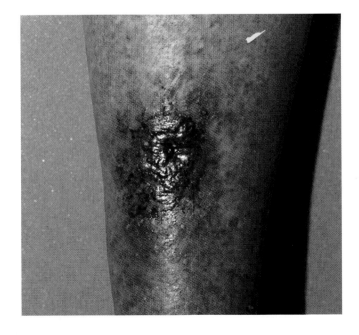

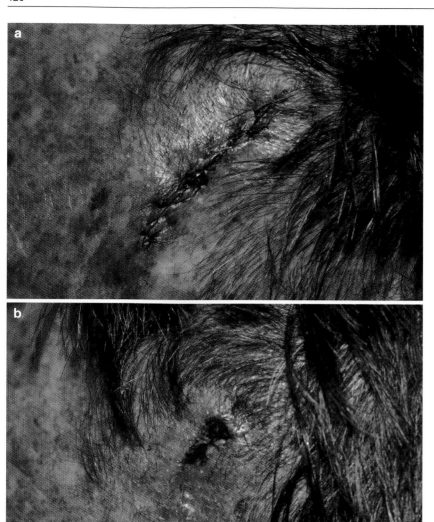

Fig. 7.5
(**a**) Sutured wound on temple.
(**b**) Dehiscence noted at 1-week post-op visit

surgery (Fig. 7.7). It is essentially a sterile abscess formed around the buried suture material. Patients often mistake this for tumor recurrence or infection. It is self-limited and tends to resolve spontaneously without a negative impact on the final cosmetic outcome. Cystic or fluctuant suture abscess can be treated with simple incision and drainage. Epidermal maturation arrest is an uncommon complication that can be problematic if it is not diagnosed. This presents as an open wound on sun-damaged skin (often scalp or forehead) that granulates in well but fails to re-epithelialize completely. There are no signs of infection and the wound bed has pink, healthy-appearing granulation tissue. The epidermis simply "stops" and does not completely cover the wound bed.

Treatment of epidermal arrest is potent topical corticosteroids. Clobetasol 0.05% ointment applied twice daily for 1–2 weeks is usually effective in bringing about complete re-epithelialization (Fig. 7.8a, b) (Jaffe et al. 1999). Use of Clobetasol should be avoided if there is exposed cartilage or bone. NSAIDS have also been reported to be effective.

Treating skin cancers requires knowledge of the potential complications. The complications covered in this chapter are not all inclusive, but cover some of the most common complications seen in the treatment of skin cancers. This knowledge will allow the practitioner to take steps to avoid these complications and to manage them once encountered.

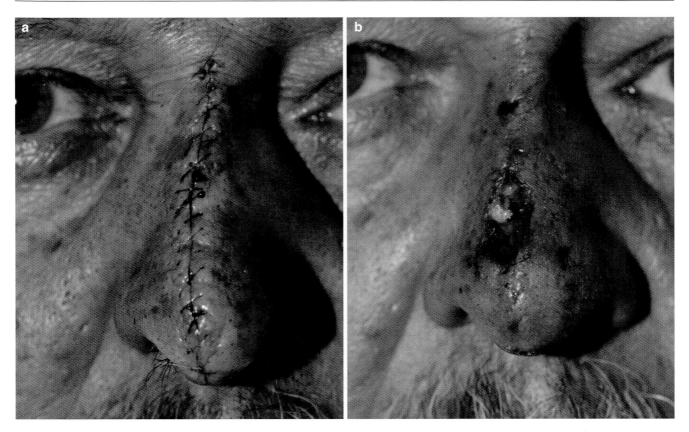

Fig. 7.6
(**a**) Sutured wound on nose. (**b**) Necrosis noted at 1-week post-op visit

Fig. 7.7
Suture granuloma on temple 4 weeks after surgery

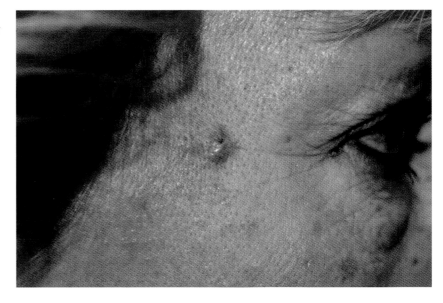

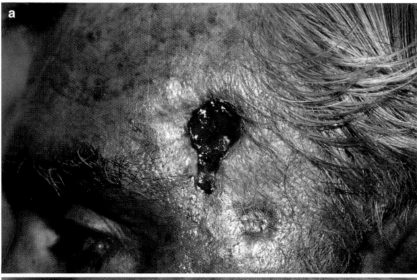

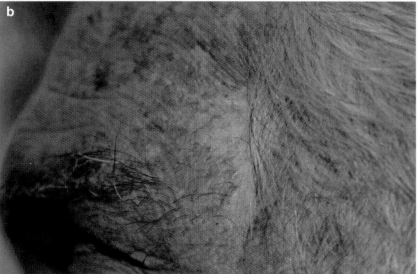

Fig. 7.8
(**a**) Open wound on temple with epidermal maturation arrest. (**b**) Complete healing after twice daily application of Class I topical steroid cream

References

Aasi S, Leffell D (2003) Complications in dermatologic surgery: how safe is safe? Arch Dermatol 139:213–214

Cook JL, Perone JB (2003) A prospective evaluation of the incidence of complications associated with Mohs micrographic surgery. Arch Dermatol 139(2):143–152

Dixon AJ, Dixon MP, Dixon JB, Del Mar CB (February 2009) Prospective study of skin surgery in smokers vs. nonsmokers. Br J Dermatol 160(2):365–367

Goldminz G, Bennett RG (1991) Cigarette smoking and flap and full-thickness graft necrosis. Arch Dermatol 127:1012–1015

Jaffe A, Heymann W, Lawrence N (1999) Epidermal maturation arrest. Dermatol Surg 25:900–903

Hendi A, Surgical complications: beyond the terrible tetrad, AAD Young Physician Focus, vol 7, No. 1, Spring 2008

Hendi A, Surgical complications: the terrible tetrad, AAD Young Physician Focus, vol 6, No. 4, Winter 2007

Index

A
Actinic keratoses (AKs), 9–13
  amelanotic melanoma, 21
  basal cell carcinoma, 18
  discoid lupus, 19–20
  hand eczema, 15
  hypertrophic actinic keratosis, 12
  lichenoid keratosis, 19
  microcystic adnexal carcinoma (MAC), 19–20
  mimickers, 13–21
  pigmented actinic keratosis, 12–13
  porokeratosis, 16
  seborrheic dermatitis, 17
  squamous cell carcinoma in situ, 16
  superficially invasive squamous cell
      carcinoma, 21
  treatment
    cryotherapy, 6–8
    topical treatments, 8
  xerosis, 14, 15
AFX. *See* Atypical fibroxanthoma
Amelanotic melanoma, 21, 81, 82
Amelonotic melanoma-invasive, 57
Amelonotic melanoma-superficial, 57
Angiofibroma, 62
Atypical fibroxanthoma (AFX), 58, 92

B
Basal cell carcinoma (BCC)
  actinic keratosis, 18
  infiltrated, chronic, 57
  infiltrative, 50, 53
  micronodular, 51
  morpheaform, 52, 54
  nodular, 50, 55
  pigmented, 54, 56
  sclerotic, 55
  treatment algorithm, 25
B cell lymphoma, 62
Benign compound nevus, 82
Benign nevi, 82
Biopsy techniques
  anatomic locations, 115
  excisional biopsy, 110–113
  incisional biopsy, 114
  local anesthesia, 99
  numbing, patient, 100–101
  punch biopsy, 106–109
  shave biopsy, 102–105
  wound care, 115
Blue nevus, 83

C
Chondrodermatitis nodularis chronica helicis (CNCH), 64
Chondrodermatitis nodularis helicis (CNH), 72
Class I topical steroid cream, 122
Congenital nevus, 83–84
Cryotherapy, 6–8
Cutaneous horn, 72
Cutaneous lupus, 61, 74
Cutaneous lymphoma, 59
Cutaneous neoplasms, 91–97

D
Dehiscence, 120
Dermatofibroma, 60
Dermatofibrosarcoma protuberans (DFSP), 58, 88, 93, 94
Dermis, skin subunits, 1
Discoid lupus, 19–20
Dysplastic nevus, 84

E
Electrodesiccation and curettage (ED&C), 27–31
EMPD. *See* Extramammary Paget's disease
Epidermal maturation arrest, 122
Epidermis, skin subunits, 1
Epithelial lining, cyst, 3
Excisional biopsy, 110–113
Extramammary Paget's disease (EMPD), 95

F
Factitial ulcers, 62, 73
Fanning technique, 33
Fibrous papule, 60
5-Fluorouracil (5-FU), 8
Follicular cyst, inflamed, 87

G
Glomus tumor, 88

H
Hand eczema, 15
Hemorrhagic blister, 86
Hydrocystoma, 91
Hypertrophic actinic keratosis, 12

I
Incisional biopsy, 114
Insect bite, 73

K
Kaposi sarcoma, 74
Keloid, 61

A. Hendi and J.C. Martinez, *Atlas of Skin Cancers*,
DOI: 10.1007/978-3-642-13399-2, © Mayo Foundation for Medical Education and Research 2011